Clinical Challenges in Paediatric Oncology

Clinical Challenges in Paediatric Oncology

Edited by

C. Ross Pinkerton

CRC Professor of Paediatric Oncology,
Department of Paediatric Oncology, Royal Marsden Hospital
and Institute of Cancer Research,
Downs Road, Sutton, UK

Antony J. Michalski

Consultant Oncologist, Department of Haematology and Oncology,
Great Ormond Street Hospital for Children, London, UK

Paul A. Veys

Bone Marrow Transplantation Consultant,
Department of Haematology and Oncology,
Great Ormond Street Hospital for Children, London, UK

I S I S
MEDICAL
MEDIA

© 1999 by Isis Medical Media Ltd.
59 St Aldates
Oxford OX1 1ST, UK

First published 1999

British Library Cataloguing in Publication Data.
A catalogue record for this title is available from
the British Library.

ISBN 1 899066 86 1

Pinkerton, C. R. (Ross)
Clinical Challenges in Paediatric Oncology
C. Ross Pinkerton, Antony J. Michalski and Paul A. Veys (eds)

Always refer to the manufacturer's Prescribing
Information before prescribing drugs cited in this book.

Page layout and typesetting
Chandos Electronic Publishing, Oxon, UK

Image reproduction
Track Direct, London, UK

Isis Medical Media staff
Publisher: Jonathan Gregory
Senior Editorial Controller: Catherine Rickards
Production Controller: Geoff Holdsworth

Printed and bound by
Book Print, S.L., Spain

Distributed in the USA by
Books International Inc., PO Box 605,
Herndon VA 20172, USA

Distributed in the rest of the world by
Plymbridge Distributors Ltd., Estover Road,
Plymouth, PL6 7PY, UK

Contents

List of contributors

Eric Bouffet
Department of Paediatric Oncology, Royal Marsden Hospital NHS Trust, Downs Road, Sutton, Surrey SM2 5PT, UK

Laurence Desjardins
Service d'onco-ophthalmologie, Institut Curie, 26 rue d'Ulm, 75248 Paris Cedex 05, France

Francois Doz
Département d'oncologie pédiatrique, Institut Curie, 26 rue d'Ulm, 75248 Paris Cedex 05, France

Nicholas Goulden
Department of Haematology and Oncology, Great Ormond Street, Hospital for Children, London WC1N 3JH, UK

Ian Hann
Department of Haematology and Oncology, Great Ormond Street, Hospital for Children, London WC1N 3JH, UK

Antony J. Michalski
Department of Haematology and Oncology, Great Ormond Street, Hospital for Children, London WC1N 3JH, UK

C. Ross Pinkerton
Department of Paediatric Oncology, Royal Marsden Hospital and Institute of Cancer Research, Downs Road, Sutton, Surrey SM2 5PT, UK

Paul A. Veys
Department of Haematology and Oncology, Great Ormond Street, Hospital for Children, London WC1N 3JH, UK

David K.H. Webb
Department of Haematology and Oncology, Great Ormond Street, Hospital for Children, London WC1N 3JH, UK

Preface

Despite major advances in recent years in the treatment of children with cancer there remain a number of important challenges. These include novel strategies to increase cure rates in those diseases where the majority of children still die and also to improve the quality of life for the growing number of long-term survivors. Great improvements have been made in the supportive care of children undergoing cancer treatment, not only in terms of medical and nursing support but also in the understanding of the psychosocial needs of these children.

Clinical Challenges in Paediatric Oncology emphasises one aspect of the multidisciplinary care of children with cancer, namely, the interaction between the oncologist, surgeon, radiotherapist, pathologist and radiologist. It focuses on some of the continuing controversies with regard to initial management and in particular the treatment strategy in the event of disease recurrence. The book is heavily illustrated and uses flow diagrams and decision trees in order to try and apply logic to these difficult situations. The text draws on the experience of authors based in two large specialist centres, namely Great Ormond Street Hospital for Children and the Royal Marsden Hospital, London. The book is intended for all those involved in the care of children with solid and haematological malignancies, both in tertiary and secondary centres. The accessibility of the text will make it a useful teaching aid for those undergoing training both in paediatric oncology and general paediatrics.

C. Ross Pinkerton

Acknowledgements

The authors are grateful to all those indirectly involved in the production of this book, namely, the departments of histopathology, diagnostic imaging and medical illustration at both the Royal Marsden Hospital and Great Ormond Street Hospital for Sick Children; in particular to Professor Richard Carter for help with pathology illustrations.

Abbreviations for treatment regimens

ATRA	all-trans retinoic acid
ABVD	doxorubicin, bleomycin, vincristine, DTIC
AraC	cytosine arabinoside
AVA	vincristine, actinomycin D, doxorubicin
BCNU	carmustine
BEAM	carmustine, etoposide, AraC, melphalan
BEP	cisplatin, etoposide, bleomycin
Bu	busulphan
CCNU	lomustine
CDDP	cisplatin
CECC	cyclophosphamide, etoposide, cyclophosphamide, carboplatin
CHOP	vincristine, cyclophosphamide, doxorubicin, prednisolone
ChlVPP	chlorambucil, vinblastine, procarbazine, prednisolone
COMP	cyclophosphamide, vincristine, low dose methotrexate, prednisolone
COPAd	cyclophosphamide, vincristine, prednisolone, doxorubicin
COPAdM-CyM	COPAd, high-dose methotrexate, cytosine
COP/COAP	cyclophosphamide, vincristine, prednisolone/doxorubicin
COPP	cyclophosphamide, vincristine, procarbazine, prednisolone
CPT-11	irinotecan
CP/Cy	cyclophosphamide
DOX	doxorubicin
EPIC	etoposide, prednisolone, ifosfamide, cisplatin
FAB LMB	Franco-American-British Lymphome Maligne Burkitt
FLAG	fludarabine, cytarabine, G-CSF
IVA	ifosfamide, vincristine, dactinomycin
IVAAd	ifosfamide, vincristine, actinomycin, doxorubicin
IVAd	ifosfamide, vincristine, doxorubicin
JEB	carboplatin, etoposide, bleomycin
LSA2 L2	vincristine, prednisone, asparaginase, daunorubicin, MTX, AraC, BCNU, hydroxyurea, mercaptopurine
MIBG	metaiodobenzylguanidine
MOPP	mustine, vinblastine, procarbazine, prednisolone, doxorubicin
MVPP	mustine, vinblastine, procarbazine, prednisolone
OJEC	vincristine, carboplatin, etoposide, cyclophosphamide
OPEC	vincristine, cisplatin, etoposide, cyclophosphamide
OPPA	vincristine, procarbazine, prednisolone, doxorubicin
PBSC	peripheral blood stem cells
PVB	cisplatin, vinblastine, bleomycin
PE CADO	cisplatin, etoposide, cyclophosphamide, doxorubicin, vincristine
PLADO	cisplatin, doxorubicin
r-tPA	recombinant tissue plasminogen activator
TBI	total body irradiation
VA	vincristine and actinomycin D
VAC	cyclophosphamide, doxorubicin, actinomycin, vincristine
VCR	vincristine

VEEP	vincristine, epirubicin, etoposide, prednisolone
VM26	teniposide
VP16	etoposide

PART I
Leukaemias and lymphomas

1

Diagnostic difficulties in paediatric acute leukaemia

2

Management of high-risk and relapsed leukaemia and indications for bone marrow transplantation

3

Complications of therapy for haematological malignancies

4

Non-Hodgkin's lymphoma

5

Hodgkin's disease

CHAPTER 1

Diagnostic difficulties in paediatric acute leukaemia

I. Hann

Introduction

The management of children with acute leukaemia is a continuing challenging problem. Diagnosis can be difficult and mistakes with this and with classification continue to be made. Overclassification (a powerful obsessional trait in some histopathologists) exerts a negative influence on thought processes and enhances prejudice. For instance, many doctors believe that acute lymphoblastic leukaemia (ALL) of T-cell origin (T-ALL) responds to different therapy than that of early B-lineage (early B-ALL) despite an almost complete lack of confirmatory evidence. However, we do know without any doubt that children with ALL of mature B-cells respond much better to intensive lymphoma-like regimens employed for ALL therapy. We also know that certain morphological subtypes of leukaemia pose life-threatening problems in supportive care, e.g. bleeding in promyelocytic leukaemia, urate nephropathy in ALL of mature B-cells, and respiratory distress syndrome (ARDS) and intracranial haemorrhage (ICH) in monocytic varieties of leukaemia.

The message must be that accurate diagnosis is essential, but overemphasis on unimportant subclassifications is detrimental and turns the mind away from important clinical entities, as well as often having no biological basis. Also, we must never make too many leaps of apparent logic. For instance, it is not true that high-risk patients will always benefit from more intensive therapy and low-risk patients do not. All risk groups of children with ALL benefit from additional intensification blocks of treatment and, for instance, high-risk patients with acute myeloid leukaemia (AML) sadly benefit little from current intensification therapy. The way to dispel such myths is to adopt a rigorous scientific approach and to use information about prognostic groupings very cautiously. After all, they only apply to the current or even retrospective series and treatment is the determinant of outcome. Adoption of risk-based strategies frequently leads to a lessening of knowledge because it is thereafter difficult to know whether therapy changes are applicable across the board or only in selected groupings.

This chapter will emphasise the errors that can be made when dealing with referred patients. Such mistakes should rarely carry any serious significance if one works within a team of experts and all cases are reviewed by several people. A doctor who ploughs his or her own furrow is guilty of arrogance and will lay themselves open to error. Nobody should treat children with leukaemia without looking at the bone marrow themselves.

It is very important to include experienced paediatric haematologists/oncologists in the management of children with leukaemia, and there is overwhelming evidence that the patients do better in the setting of a children's cancer centre. When a patient presents to a centre with possible leukaemia, the classical approach is to take a good history, carry out a thorough clinical examination, then look at the blood count and blood film and then to proceed to lumbar puncture (LP) and the crucial diagnostic test, a bone marrow aspirate. This approach will be mirrored in the text below and will incorporate newer diagnostic tests such as those using monoclonal antibodies and molecular biology testing. These tests are gradually replacing the need for older technologies such as bone marrow cytochemistry and classical cytogenetics. They lead the way to less subjective diagnostic techniques and point the way towards aetiological mechanisms, but there is a real and present danger of throwing out the 'baby with the bathwater'. Overinterpretation of such tests and failure to maintain a holistic approach to diagnosis leads to error. Simple bone marrow morphology remains the most crucial aspect of diagnosis.

Clinical history

Acute leukaemia can occur at any age in childhood, although the gender and age can give clues as to the diagnosis. T-cell leukaemia is uncommon in girls and ALL presents mainly between the ages of 2 and 5 years. Young infants with leukaemia may have ALL or AML and it is important to look for symptoms and signs of central nervous system (CNS) disease and other extramedullary disease, e.g. in the gums and skin, because it is more common in the very young. Patients with Down's syndrome should be managed with caution when very young because they are prone to transient abnormal myelopoiesis (TAM) and leukaemoid reactions (Figs. 1.1 and 1.2), which can be mistaken for true leukaemia (Table 1.1).

A clinical history (Box 1.1) provides the basic framework upon which examinations leading to diagnosis are based.

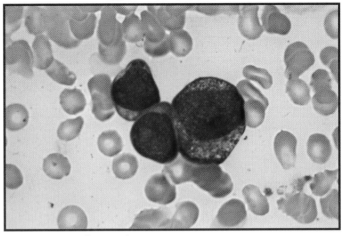

Figure 1.2 *Leukaemoid reactions.*

Box 1.1 Clinical history

Symptoms:
  Bone pain
  Breathlessness
  Upper limb and neck swelling
  Febrile episodes
  Bruising/purpura
  Anorexia
Family history:
  Fanconi anaemia
  Bloom's syndrome
  Shwachman syndrome
  Neurofibromatosis
  Other children with leukaemia: identical twins, myelodysplasia
Drugs:
  e.g. aspirin, sodium valproate, phenytoin, cimetidine
Recent past history:
  Bleeding, e.g. epistaxes
  Infections
  Contact with infections, e.g. chicken pox
  Growth impaired
  Travel abroad

Symptoms

Presenting symptoms in children with leukaemia relate to the marrow infiltration or expansion and the consequent marrow failure, along with deposition of leukaemic cells in the reticuloendothelial system and sometimes in the CNS, testes, ovaries, kidneys, retinae, skin and gums. Detectable extramedullary disease is

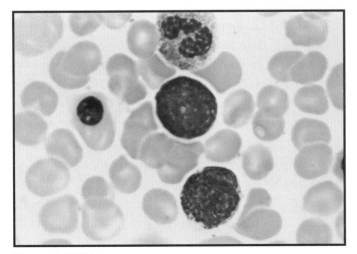

Figure 1.1 *TAM.*

Table 1.1 Differential diagnosis of acute leukaemia

Symptom/sign	Differential causes	Examples
Pancytopenias	Infections	Tuberculosis and MAI; leishmaniasis; SBE; CMV; meningococcaemia; severe and overwhelming infections; EBV; HIV; hepatitis
	Haemophagocytic lymphohistiocytosis (HLH)	Familial; viral-induced; idiopathic; leukaemia-associated
	Marrow failure	Aplastic anemia; Shwachman syndrome; Pearson syndrome; Fanconi anaemia
	Marrow infiltration	Neuroblastoma; other tumours, e.g. rhabdomyosarcoma
Isolated cytopenias	Platelets	ITP; drugs; WAS; HUS; TTP; DIC; Bernard–Soulier syndrome; Kasabach–Merrit syndrome
	Anaemias	Haemolytic; congenital dyserythropoietic anaemia; sideroblastic anaemia; Diamond–Blackfan anaemia
	Neutropenias	Kostman syndrome; others
(Hepato)splenomegaly	Infections	Tuberculosis and MAI; leishmaniasis; SBE; CMV; meningococcaemia; severe and overwhelming infections; EBV; HIV; hepatitis
	Storage diseases	
	Metabolic diseases	
	Haemophagocytic lymphohistiocytosis	
	Osteopetrosis	
	Liver problems	Hepatic fibrosis
	Malaria	
	Chronic myeloid leukaemia	
	Lymphomas	
	Other myeloproliferative disorders and myelodysplasias	Essential thrombocythaemia
Bone pain and bone changes	Autoimmune and rheumatoid diseases	
	Tumours	Neuroblastoma
	Osteomyelitis	
Purpura/petechiae/ bleeding	Coagulation disorders	
	Protein C deficiency	
	Meningococcaemia	
	Non-accidental injury	

CMV, cytomegalovirus; DIC, disseminated intravascular coagulation; EBV, Epstein–Barr virus; HUS, haemolytic–uraemic syndrome; ITP, idiopathic thrombocytopenic purpura; MAI, *Mycobacterium avium-intracellulare* infection; SBE, subacute bacterial endocarditis; TTP, thrombotic thrombocytopenic purpura; WAS, Wiskott–Aldrich syndrome.

quite uncommon at diagnosis, even though the disease is obviously widespread in all cases at the outset.

Bone marrow infiltration and expansion leads to bone pain in about two-thirds of patients. In the past, extensive radiology was performed in all cases of leukaemia at diagnosis. This is no longer justified (other than routine chest X-ray to look for mediastinal mass) because it does not alter clinical management. Many children with leukaemia were treated for suspected rheumatoid disorders in the past, but X-ray examination rarely helps to identify these and there is now a much greater awareness of the need to examine such patients with aches and pains carefully, to look for organomegaly and assiduously to examine the blood film and blood count.

Bone marrow failure leads to anaemia, which in children frequently presents as lethargy, irritability, anorexia, pallor and, occasionally, breathlessness. Lack of good functioning white cells renders these patients susceptible to febrile episodes before and after diagnosis. Lack of platelets often leads to skin and mucosal purpura and petechiae and, rarely, to haemorrhages in the optic fundi. The fundi must, however, always be rigorously examined because blindness can be prevented by judicious use of platelets and possibly other coagulation factors. Patients with a mediastinal mass usually develop varying degrees of superior vena cava (SVC) obstruction, which can be life threatening and lead to upper limb and neck oedema along with obstruction of the upper airways. Such patients must never be placed in positions that compromise the airways. For instance, curling them up in order to perform a lumbar puncture may lead to respiratory arrest. Urgent diagnosis is essential in these patients.

Family history

Certain genetic disorders such as Down's syndrome predispose children to leukaemia. Within the family history and clinical examination, it is also necessary to rule out other predisposition syndromes such as Fanconi anaemia and Bloom's syndrome, which are DNA repair defects usually presenting with bone marrow aplasia, sometimes later evolving into acute leukaemia. Rare families with AML and myelodysplasia may contain several affected children, and this may be associated with platelet storage pool defects.

Drugs

Taking a comprehensive history of drug ingestion should be part of the initial process of any child's clinical administration, but it rarely adds greatly to the management of children with leukaemia. It does, however, help to identify causes of cytopenias not resulting from leukaemia but rather from failures of cell production. For instance, children with epilepsy may be taking drugs like phenytoin, which can lead to thrombocytopenia.

Recent past history

Quite often the child will have had more infections than usual over the preceding several months and parents may feel that they can pinpoint a time of onset for the leukaemia. There is often a gradual downhill course but, more rarely, a very acute onset can occur. Weight loss may have been noted, which may be in excess of that expected for the level of existing anorexia. It is important at this stage to enquire about infectious contact and foreign travel. Children who have recently been in contact with chicken pox (varicella–zoster) infection may be in the incubation period and can go on to develop severe infections when treatment is started if adequate prophylaxis with zoster immunoglobulin is not given promptly. When initially considering the differential diagnosis (Table 1.1) it may help to directly enquire about countries recently visited. Children with leishmaniasis may present with hepatosplenomegaly, weight loss and pancytopenia, resembling acute leukaemia. Such a case was initially missed because the parents were asked about 'exotic' holidays and did not think that Spanish and Mediterranean holidays were particularly exotic! It is always important to be sure that one is not dealing with infections or autoimmune disorders when investigating a blood dyscrasia.

Clinical examination

Having taken the clinical history, the physical examination usually gives the major clues to the diagnosis and is of vital importance (Box 1.2). For instance, if you have a patient before you with obvious bruising and anaemia then you should be considering bone marrow hypoplasia and leukaemia as the most

---

Box 1.2 Clinical examination

Signs of bleeding

Signs of anaemia

Lymphadenopathy

Hepatosplenomegaly

Wasting

Optic fundi

Joints/bone

Skin

Infections

Cranial nerves

Tissue deposits in other sites: testes, gums, ovaries, retina

Chest

---

likely cause. Liver and/or spleen enlargement are common in leukaemia and rare in marrow hypoplasia disorders. Clearly this is not a hard and fast rule because a small proportion of children with leukaemia do not have hepatosplenomegaly and there are, of course, other causes, such as haemophagocytic lymphohistiocytosis (HLH), various infections especially in early infancy and liver problems.

Signs of bleeding

As stated above, marrow failure caused by production failure or marrow hypoplasia usually leads to anaemia, neutropenia and thrombocytopenia. In addition to the low level of platelets, children with leukaemia may also have abnormalities of the coagulation proteins resulting from liver dysfunction and/or disseminated intravascular coagulation (DIC), usually consequent upon infections. The majority of patients will present with cutaneous petechiae and bruising, sometimes along with mucosal bleeding and, occasionally, bleeding in the optic fundi. It is, therefore, particularly important to look in the mouth and optic fundi of all patients presenting with a bleeding disorder because urgent therapy to preserve sight and prevent more serious bleeding may be indicated.

Whenever such symptoms or signs are present it is essential to check the platelet count and blood film along with a prothrombin time (PT), partial thromboplastin time (PTT) and fibrinogen level. If these prove to be normal and the platelet count is not very low, then a bleeding time will help to rule out thrombasthenia, prior to platelet aggregation and von Willebrand factor tests.

Signs of anaemia

Most patients who present with leukaemia have a compensated anaemia, because there is a slow fall in red blood cells owing to failure of production. Severe and rapid falls in haemoglobin levels should alert one to causes related to consumption (DIC, haemolytic–uraemic syndrome [HUS], HLH, Evans' syndrome of autoimmune haemolysis and thrombocytopenia), or bleeding. The signs of anaemia are usually just pallor and lethargy, although occasionally one can hear a heart gallop rhythm or detect hepatomegaly and tachycardia because of heart failure.

Lymphadenopathy

Most children with leukaemia have some lymph node enlargement and the most frequent diagnostic difficulty is differentiating normal childhood adenopathy from more sinister causes. In clinical practice, this is a very common problem and very frequently perfectly normal children present to clinics with small neck nodes and nothing else apart from a recent history of upper respiratory and/or ear infections. In almost every case, the only real problem is usually anxiety, which can be extreme and often exacerbated by medical staff. Formal guidelines on how to manage such patients are inappropriate. Indeed, guidelines are becoming something of a modern curse! In their place, they are invaluable but they have major drawbacks because they tend to stifle thought and waste resources through development of poorly thought out lists of tests. There is no substitute for clinical acumen and this is one of the most important areas in which it should be applied. The clues for a benign cause are glands that are not very big and not increasing in size, that are smooth and mobile and may be associated with recent local infection and that occur in a generally well child with no hepatosplenomegaly. The clues for malignancy are basically the opposite, along with signs of anaemia, petechiae or purpura and general ill-health. If in doubt, check the blood count and blood film and maybe check a chest X-ray film for mediastinal mass.

Always remember that a diagnosis made a few days or few weeks earlier very rarely makes the slightest difference in a well child. *Confident* reassurance to wait and watch is often all that is required. 'Reassurance' biopsies are not in the interests of the child and must be avoided.

Hepatosplenomegaly

It is very important to examine the abdomen well. That sounds like a trite and obvious statement, but organomegaly is still frequently missed because an upset child is examined in a hurry. The investment of time spent in calming down and properly examining children in this situation is well spent. When one finds hepatosplenomegaly then it is usually the case that it is necessary to institute a panel of investigations including a bone marrow aspirate in order to define the problem. In the UK, the most common cause of splenomegaly with or without hepatomegaly is probably a Budd–Chiari syndrome variant seen after neonatal catheterisation and liver disease, such as hepatic fibrosis. In other parts of the world, infections would be far commoner, including malaria, leishmaniasis, amoebiasis, etc. In these situations, the blood picture is usually one of hypersplenism, in which there is moderate thrombocytopenia, mild anaemia and moderate leucopenia with no excess of abnormal forms on the blood film. At this stage, it is usual to institute a thorough search for infectious causes such as cytomegalovirus (CMV) and Epstein–Barr virus (EBV) infection and possibly for human immunodeficiency virus (HIV) if the blood film does not give any clues; these can occur while proceeding to bone marrow aspiration.

There are a number of other rarer diseases that produce hepatosplenomegaly, but these do not usually produce any abnormalities in the blood count and are associated with classical clinical features. In a very young child, in particular, it is always very important to rule out metabolic diseases, which usually present in a sick child with obvious metabolic problems. Storage diseases usually present in the young with cerebral and other organ dysfunction and some can be diagnosed from the blood film or bone marrow and physical examination. One disease that is sometimes initially misdiagnosed is osteopetrosis, which does produce a leukaemia-like (leukaemoid) blood film, and this is one diagnosis that should never be forgotten in the very young.

Wasting

Children with leukaemia lose weight because of anorexia and probably because of excessive production of cachexins. In any child with growth failure, one should think of the bone marrow failure syndromes such as Fanconi anaemia and Shwachman's syndrome, the diagnosis being obvious following bone marrow examination, which will show reduced or dysplastic cellularity but no excess of leukaemic blast cells in the early stages.

Optic fundi

Nowadays there is a tendency for patients to present at a much earlier stage and it is, therefore, uncommon to see extensive haemorrhage and leukaemic infiltration in the optic fundi (Fig. 1.3a). This can still be seen sometimes in patients with a very high white blood cell count (WBC) at diagnosis and at CNS relapse and in patients with promyelocytic leukaemia. In rare cases, there can be doubt over the diagnosis, for example patients with CMV infection may have similar optic changes. Tapping of the aqueous humor with cytospin examination is usually diagnostic where a hypopion exists, but otherwise the diagnosis rests on the usual cerebrospinal fluid (CSF) cytospin and bone marrow examination (Fig. 1.3.b).

It is also very important to look for papilloedema because a small percentage of patients with ALL and monocytic varieties of AML present with CNS disease at diagnosis: a brain computerised tomography (CT) or magnetic resonance imaging (MRI) scan should be performed before lumbar puncture in such cases, but nearly always there is no obstructive cause and the hydrocephalus is communicating.

Joints and bone

Bone pain occurs in about two-thirds of patients with leukaemia and can be very severe; it is sometimes associated with local tenderness. More usually, there is generalised tenderness or irritability, which improves rapidly after anti-leukaemia therapy is started. In the past, patients with leukaemia were often labelled as having 'growing pains' or 'irritable' hip or nebulous rheumatoid disorders. This mistake rarely occurs

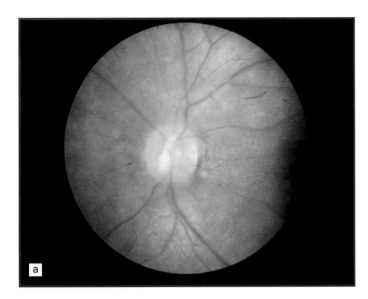

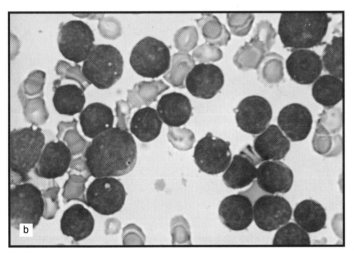

Figure 1.3 *(a) Optic fundus infiltrated by meningeal leukaemia; (b) CSF cytospin.*

nowadays but we continue to see occasional patients who are treated with steroids; this masks the true diagnosis because about half of the children with ALL will have a temporary remission with this therapy. It is essential to be especially careful when giving therapy, particularly potentially dangerous drugs like steroids, for such diseases that are diagnosed by exclusion.

Skin
Other than cutaneous bleeding, the examination of the skin rarely helps in the diagnosis. In young babies, subcutaneous lumps may be the first sign of leukaemia. In older children (particularly with pre-B ALL) this does occasionally occur and is characteristic of Ki-1 lymphomas. If a very young child has eczema and thrombocytopenia, this should immediately alert one to Wiskott–Aldrich syndrome (WAS), especially if infections have been a problem. A genetic test for this disorder is now available.

Children with autoimmune disorders may have rashes that are vasculitic in nature or look like erythema nodosum, and which tend to involve the face (cheeks). Finally, one should always look for cutaneous manifestations of infection, which may be the primary problem (e.g. toxoplasmosis) or interfere with therapy for leukaemia (e.g. chicken pox).

Cranial nerves
Palsies of cranial nerves rarely occur at the outset of leukaemia treatment although VII cranial nerve abnormalities in the absence of other evidence of CNS leukaemia may resolve with standard ALL-type therapy. More characteristically, patients with ALL of mature B-cell phenotype can occasionally present with cranial nerve palsies. MRI is often performed but rarely contributes any useful information.

Tissue deposits/other organs
One of the difficult differential diagnoses can be with Stage 4 neuroblastoma in which marrow may be replaced by malignant cells that can look like lymphoblasts and that do not always conveniently form into clumps or rosettes. Examination of the abdomen may help to identify the primary tumour. Leukaemia of mature B-cells very often presents with multiple large abdominal masses, sometimes including ovarian masses, which are very uncommon in other types of leukaemia. Other sites are infrequently involved, but testes can be involved at diagnosis in ALL and gums can be infiltrated in congenital and monocytic varieties of leukaemia.

Chest
Examination of the chest is obligatory, firstly to rule out infection, this being one of the commonest presenting sites and, secondly, in order to diagnose superior vena cava obstruction, which usually necessitates very urgent diagnosis and therapy. In fact, anaesthesia for these patients is very difficult to perform safely, and performing lumbar puncture may well lead to respiratory arrest and should be avoided until the situation is more stable (Fig. 1.4). The usual

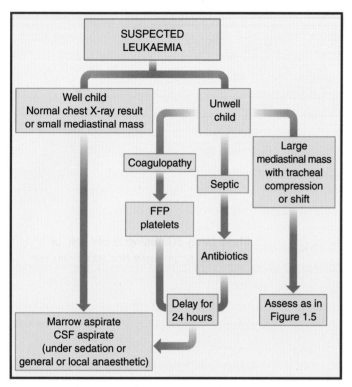

Figure 1.4 *Algorithm for assessment of a child with suspected leukaemia.*

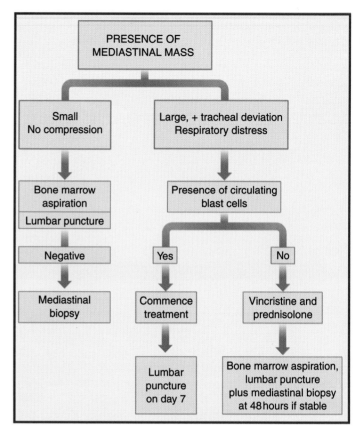

Figure 1.5 *Algorithm for assessment of a child with a mediastinal mass.*

approach is to look at the blood film and, if it is normal and there is concern about the tolerability of anaesthesia or sedation, to commence therapy with vincristine and steroids, along with forced diuresis because of the risk of urate nephropathy. A diagnostic biopsy can be done once the tumour has shrunk and the patient's condition is stable (Fig. 1.5).

Patients who have mature B-cell ALL often have large pleural effusions and in the absence of bone marrow disease a diagnosis can sometimes be made from a pleural aspirate by the presence of L3 lymphoblasts with clonal surface membrane immunoglobulin.

Investigations

When the patient arrives through the door there are two types of test that must be performed: those required to check for organ dysfunction or potential clinical problems and those required for diagnosis (Table 1.2). People should not be investigated by lists, because that is the perfect way to make mistakes and waste precious resources. The tests should be step-wise and tailored to the initial findings. Thereafter, they

should be designed to identify the important classification and prognostic subgroups that hopefully are of real clinical value and not simply part of a 'stamp-collecting' exercise.

The full blood count and blood film

The most important first test, which should be available everywhere, is a full blood count and blood film, looked at by somebody who regularly sees films from children and those with leukaemia. In many cases, it will then be obvious that the patient has leukaemia, and the only remaining problem will be in deciding on its subclassification into various myeloid and lymphoid subtypes, which requires that a bone marrow aspirate be performed. The problems that arise at this stage are often caused by worries about what used to be called 'aleukaemic leukaemia', where there are various cytopenias but no obvious blast cells on a blood film, which happens in about one in ten patients. The other problem occurs when the blood contains non-leukaemic blast cells that are produced because they spill out from the marrow. Typical situations would be the so-called 'stressed neonate',

Table 1.2 Obligatory investigations in cases of acute leukaemia		
Investigation	Subgroups	Use
Blood tests	Full blood count and blood film	Diagnosis and classification of leukaemia into subgroups; differential diagnosis
	Coagulation screen	Hepatic disease, infection
	Blood group, crossmatch and direct Coombs' test	Evans' syndrome, autoimmune disorders
	Urea, electrolytes, urate, liver function tests	Urate nephropathy, hepatic disease
Chest X-ray		Assessing infection and mediastinal mass Anterior mass usually T-ALL or T-cell non-Hodgkin's lymphoma (T-NHL)
		Mass rarely sclerosing; B-cell NHL or teratoma, sometimes Hodgkin's disease
Lumbar puncture	Cytospin	Malignant cells; differential diagnosis
Bone marrow	Morphology	Definitive test
	Cytochemical stain: Sudan Black, PAS and acid phosphatase usually enough; if possibility of monocytic leukaemia, also do NSE	
	Immunophenotype: minimum panel is CD10, CD19, CD13, CD33, tdt, CD2, CD7; add glycophorin if possibly erythroid; add CD41 plus CD61 if possibly megakaryoblastic	
	Marrow cytogenetics and DNA ploidy	

NSE, non-specific esterase; PAS, periodic acid Schiff stain.

occasional children with a leukoerythroblastic reaction to infection and children with marrow infiltration, e.g. osteopetrosis, neuroblastoma. In addition, transient abnormal myelopoiesis (TAM) may present in this way.

Other blood tests

Liver function tests should be performed because a rare patient may present with severe hepatic problems presumably caused by infiltration of that organ, as there is usually no indication of viral hepatitis. Urea, creatinine and blood electrolytes should be checked because of the risk of urate nephropathy, which may be present even from diagnosis; the highest risk patients are those with leukaemia of mature B-cells and those with a mediastinal mass, but any patient with a high WBC at diagnosis (usually greater than 100×10^9 cells/l) is at high-risk. Checking renal and hepatic function will also rule out other causes of cytopenia without blast cells, for instance HUS, which usually but not always presents with dramatic

red cell fragmentation on the blood film, which is called microangiopathic haemolytic anaemia (MAHA).

It is probably also wise to check a coagulation screen and fibrinogen degradation products because some patients will have developed liver dysfunction coagulopathy and others DIC, related usually to infection. It may be necessary, therefore, to use coagulation product replacement as well as platelet transfusions. We have also seen one patient with subacute bacterial endocarditis (SBE) who presented with severe pancytopenia owing to marrow suppression and DIC, along with hepatosplenomegaly.

The only other important blood test is the blood group and cross-match with direct Coombs' test. Patients with autoimmune haemolytic anaemia (AIHA) and thrombocytopenia, which is called Evans' syndrome, usually present in early infancy with anaemia and low platelets. Also, patients with cytopenias caused by autoimmune disorders often have a positive direct Coombs' test.

X-ray examination

The only routinely useful test is a chest X-ray, which will help to pick up tracheal deviation or obstruction caused by a mediastinal mass as well as pleural effusions (Fig. 1.5). In addition, occult chest infections can occur prior to diagnosis and should lead to intensive efforts to secure a specific diagnosis. Other radiology is infrequently of value, although it would be wise to X-ray bones that are particularly painful or show any signs of fracture, which happens rarely. A small proportion of patients have severe extensive spinal osteoporosis and collapsed vertebral bodies, which usually heal adequately with anti-leukaemic therapy alone. The presence of cranial nerve palsies or optic involvement should lead to MRI or CT brain scanning.

Lumbar puncture

A cytospin of CSF is required from every patient who has leukaemia, because the presence of CNS disease at diagnosis alters the management policy thereafter. It may also be helpful in the differential diagnosis of diseases that cause meningitis, such meningo-coccaemia, and other diseases affecting the CNS such as HLH, which may produce a moderate pleocytosis of phagocytosing macrophages.

Bone marrow examination

Bone marrow aspiration is the crucial test that will usually give the diagnosis and besides which most other results should be regarded as merely confirmatory (Fig. 1.6). Some patients with bone marrow fibrosis (myelofibrosis) have marrows that are so scarred that it is impossible to aspirate a satisfactory sample from the usual sites, e.g. the iliac crests. In such instances, it is rarely, if ever, justified to try other and much more dangerous sites such as the sternum and tibia, which in any case hardly ever yield better samples. Repeat attempts at aspiration along with a good marrow trephine biopsy should be carried out. It must always be remembered that myelofibrosis is a description and not a proper diagnosis, and that acute myelofibrosis is extremely rare in children. However, dramatic fibrosis is associated with megakaryoblastic leukaemia, as a result of the production of fibrosis-producing platelet-derived growth factor (PDGF). Other causes include tuberculosis, toxoplasmosis, HIV,

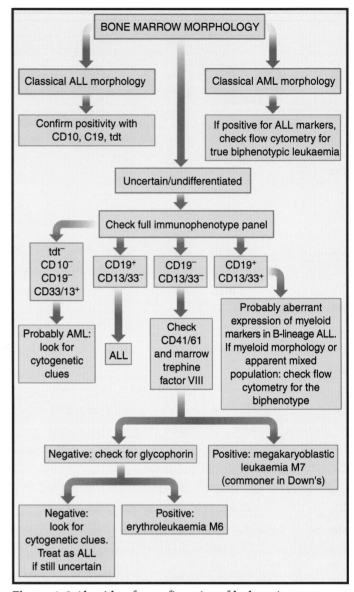

Figure 1.6 *Algorithm for confirmation of leukaemia type.*

Tγ-lymphoproliferative disease, myeloproliferative disorders, ALL (10% of cases), AML and autoimmune disorders.

Common cytochemical stains

Two cytochemical stains are the mainstay of diagnosis, being the iron stain and May–Grünwald–Giemsa (MGG) or its equivalent. The iron stain will pick up cases of sideroblastic anaemia, myelodysplasia with ringed sideroblasts and Pearson's syndrome which is also associated with cytoplasmic vacuolation and metabolic disorders.

The MGG stain is first examined for cellularity and, therefore, it should immediately split the diagnosis into failures of production, or hypoplasia, and proliferative disorders. This enables the hypoplastic anaemias to be ruled out, which include: aplastic anaemia, Fanconi anaemia, dyskeratosis congenita, Shwachman syndrome, Diamond–Blackfan anaemia and Kostman syndrome. In the last two, the overall cellularity may be normal but there is a deficiency of normoblasts in the first and late granulocytes in the latter.

Secondly, one should search for storage cells such as Gaucher cells, Nieman–Pick cells and sea-blue histiocytes. Also, on low-power examination, one can usually see inclusion bodies especially those of Leishman–Donovan bodies and Chediak–Higashi inclusions. Other infections like filaria can be seen and tuberculosis should be investigated by immunological methods in addition to Ziehl–Neelsen staining. At low power, clumps of malignant cells should be obvious and this is a common finding in Stage 4 neuroblastoma. Infiltrates from non-Hodgkin's lymphoma (NHL) are identical to a low-level infiltrate of leukaemia and are nearly always associated with high-stage and high-grade disease elsewhere. Otherwise, any malignant infiltrate is uncommon in children and usually restricted to rhabdomyosarcoma, Ewing's tumour, Hodgkin's disease and Langerhans cell histiocytosis.

The finding of a normal marrow is compatible with certain immune disorders such as idiopathic thrombocytopenic purpura (ITP), although sometimes there appears to be an excess of megakaryocytes. Other immune disorders such as systemic lupus erythematosis (SLE) and dermatomyositis can present with some degree of dysplasia along with haemophagocytic macrophages identical in appearance to HLH, and myelofibrosis. The diagnosis of HLH depends on the finding of phagocytic macrophages in the bone marrow, which are ingesting particularly red cells and platelets, and occasionally WBC. This most often occurs in young children, with hepatosplenomegaly, fevers and pancytopenia. It can occur in older children and may be associated with viral infections, particularly EBV.

Patients with myelodysplasia and myeloproliferative disorders usually present with a hypercellular marrow, although cellularity can sometimes be reduced. The essential features of most cases are dysplastic changes with hypogranulation, irregular or abnormal nuclei and abnormal size with megaloblastic change. The iron stain may show ringed sideroblasts. An increasing proportion of blast cells in the marrow indicates one of the disorders that usually leads on to myeloid leukaemia in children. Roughly speaking the classification is: refractory anaemia <5% blast cells; refractory anaemia with excess blast cells 5 to 10/15%; refractory anaemia with excess of blast cells in transformation, 15–25% blast cells. The prominent dysplasia, which is often even more dramatic on the blood film, usually gives the game away and chromosome changes, especially monosomy 7, may also help. Of the myeloproliferative disorders in children, the most common is juvenile myelomonocytic leukaemia (JMML), which can be associated with high haemoglobin F levels, monosomy of chromosome 7 and a blood monocytosis. Persistent excess of platelets (essential thrombocythaemia) is very rare in children and there is usually an excess of marrow megakaryocytes. Persistent dramatic eosinophilia is also very rare and chromosome 5 abnormalities in the region of the interleukin-5 (IL-5) gene may be seen. Chronic myeloid leukaemia (CML) also only accounts for about 2 in 100 of leukaemias in children and the Philadelphia chromosome and *bcr/abl* or *abl/bcr* proto-oncogenes will be found in the blood or marrow. Although there is hepatosplenomegaly and sometimes blast cells in the blood, the give-away is the cytogenetic finding along with a very high blood WBC, consisting mainly of early myeloid cells in all stages of maturation.

Special cytochemical stains

Specialized cytochemical stains for bone marrow aspirates are becoming progressively less necessary as time goes by. However, in those parts of the world where immunophenotyping and cytogenetics are not readily available, they still can be useful. Also, they allow a 'belt and braces' approach, which sometimes helps in classification of leukaemias (Figs. 1.7 and 1.8). To put it simply, and there is no longer any justification to make it complicated, ALL cases are usually periodic acid–Schiff (PAS) positive and Sudan Black (SB) negative. T-cell ALL cases usually show block positivity with the acid phosphatase stain in the position of the Golgi apparatus. Myeloid leukaemias

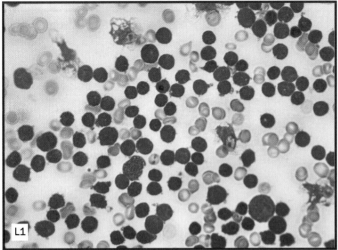

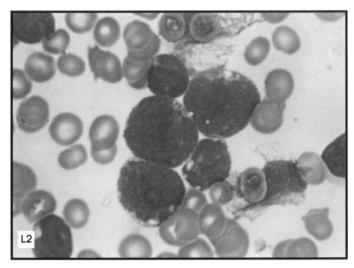

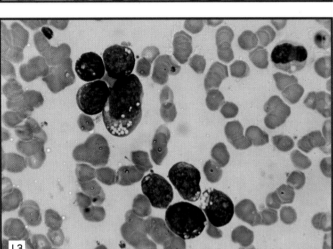

Figure 1.7 *Morphological classification and relevance in ALL.*
L1. Microlymphoblastic acute leukaemia. Usually more than 75% of cells are small with non-prominent nucleoli, high nucleo-cytoplasmic ratio and little nuclear folding. Cells tend to be periodic acid–Schiff (PAS) positive. No clinical significance.
L2. Macrolymphoblastic leukaemia. Usually more than 75% of cells are large, often with prominent nucleoli, nuclear folding and abundant cytoplasm.
L3. Cells of this type are almost always associated with mature B-cell (surface membrane immunoglobulin-positive) ALL. Beware vacuolated L2 cases, which can look similar but have less basophilic cytoplasm (if the staining is adequate) and are surface immunoglobulin-negative. This is a very important diagnosis because these patients are at very high-risk of urate nephropathy and often require dialysis. They also require different therapy and do very badly with straightforward ALL therapy and well with lymphoma-like regimens.

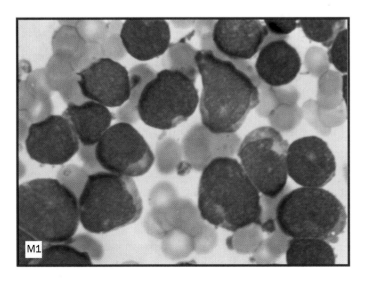

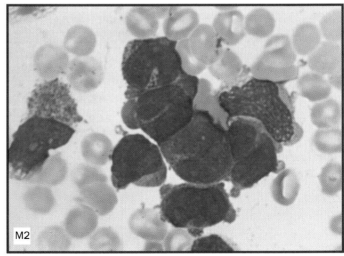

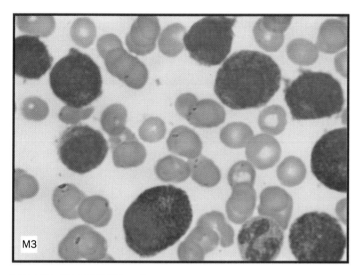

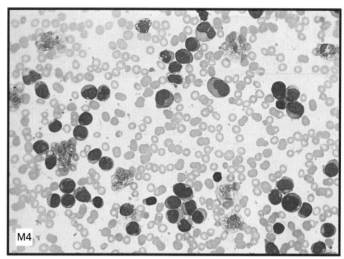

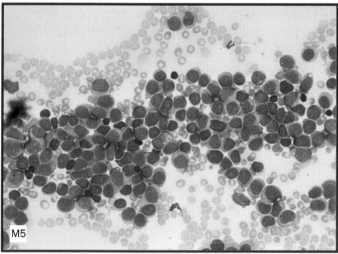

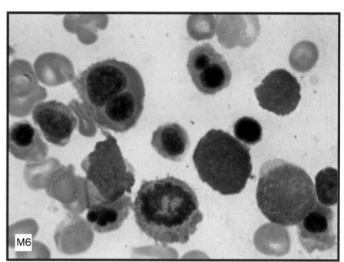

Figure 1.8 *Morphological classification in AML and clinical relevance.*

M1. Undifferentiated AML. Some myeloid differentiation occurs with granulated blasts. Often positive for Sudan Black stain.

M2. Differentiated AML. Differentiated myeloid occurs with prominent granules and usually Auer rods; positive for staining with Sudan Black. This stage has a good prognosis; patients with t(8;21) usually have this variety.

M3. Promyelocytic leukaemia. These patients have abnormalities of the retinoic acid receptor gene t(15;17) and a good prognosis. However, they get DIC and should be treated from the outset with all-trans-retinoic acid. Beware high rises in WBC on this treatment as it can lead to pulmonary and other problems, so start cytotoxics early.

M4. Myelomonocytic leukaemia.

M5. Monocytic and monoblastic leukaemia. Both M4 and M5 types have a tendency to high WBC counts and extramedullary disease, e.g. gums, skin, CNS. Beware problems of leukostasis, especially ARDS and ICH.

M6. Erythroid leukaemia. This is very rare in children. Beware mixing up with dyserythropoietic anaemias. JMML may have a prominent erythroid element.

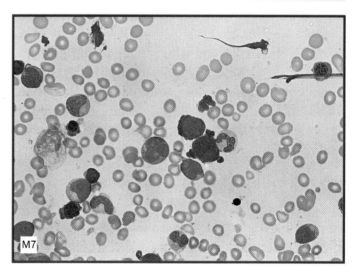

M7. Megakaryoblastic leukaemia. This is often associated with Down's syndrome. It may present with osteosclerosis. The marrow is often very difficult to aspirate because of myelofibrosis. Down's patients do very well without BMT.

are usually SB positive and PAS negative, with especially strong staining in the promyelocytic variety (M3). However, there is an important catch here in that there is a form of promyelocytic leukaemia that is hypogranular and the diagnosis depends on identifying the 'cottage-loaf' nuclear forms and the t(15;17) translocation (Fig. 1.9). As already stated, this is an important diagnosis because early therapy with *all-trans*-retinoic acid abrogates the bleeding problem.

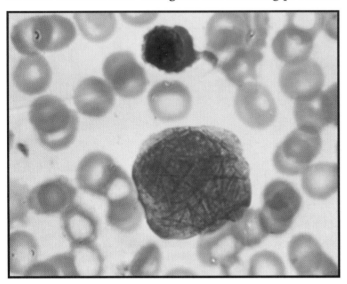

Figure 1.9 *'Cottage-loaf' nuclei, with Auer rods.*

In other forms of myeloid leukaemia, these stains can also produce useful information. The monocytic varieties are usually diffusely positive with non-specific esterase (NSE) stain and with acid phosphatase. These patients have a tendency to early CNS disease, hyperleukocytosis and consequent leukostasis. Erythroid leukaemias are usually block or granular positive with PAS and megakaryoblastic leukaemias are usually NSE positive.

Immunophenotyping

The monoclonal antibody tests provide useful confirmatory information and have helped to classify almost all acute leukaemias into lymphoid and myeloid categories. The antibodies are considerably more useful in ALL than in AML and, as shown in Tables 1.2 and 1.3, it is possible to classify ALL along the lines of the normal lymphoid ontogenetic pathway. When differentiating AML from ALL in childhood, the former are rarely terminal deoxynucleotidyl transferase

(tdt) positive and also rarely positive with CD10 or CD19. Occasional positivity is seen with T-cell antigens, which may indicate a truly biphenotypic leukaemia or possibly just aberrant expression. The latter has little prognostic importance, whereas the former is a very rare situation leading to a poor prognosis. In these cases, it is very helpful to look at cell sorter scans to see whether the paradoxical antigens are expressed on separate cells. In situations of doubt, it is usually best to treat the most likely morphological type (mainly ALL) and follow progress, because AML will declare itself if it is lurking there.

The biggest mistake with immunophenotyping is to look at it in isolation from the rest of the findings. To put it crudely, if the immunophenotyping does not make sense in itself or if it does not correlate with the morphology, then the phenotyping is usually wrong. The commonest mistake is to take too much notice of so-called myeloid antigens CD13 and CD33, which are frequently co-expressed on B-lineage leukaemias. Also, to take too much notice of CD10 and tdt results in marrows with low blast cell proportions, because this often happens in normal children and those with infection, neutropenia, Diamond–Blackfan anaemia, etc.

Immunophenotyping does have its place and one of them is to confirm the diagnosis of leukaemia of mature B-cells when clonal surface membrane immunoglobulin is positive. This is helpful, because these patients need lymphoma-like treatment and are at very high-risk of urate nephropathy.

Genetic tests

Classical cytogenetic testing is gradually losing its value and is being superseded by the new DNA technologies. This technology will be useful for prognostic purposes and there are already suggestions that counting chromosomes can be replaced by DNA ploidy testing, which can detect hyperdiploid clones of very good prognosis and near-haploid clones of very poor prognosis. This is also helpful for diagnosis and can be supplemented by the cytogenetic tests for the changes shown in Tables 1.4 and 1.5. However, such tests are rarely necessary and some continue to take too long to be useful in this situation. A useful algorithm for confirmation of leukaemia type is given in Figure 1.6.

Table 1.3 Typical pattern of antigen expression according to cell lineage					
Marker	B-lineage	T-lineage	Myeloid	Megakaryocytic	Erythroid
CD45	+	+	–	+	+
CD19[a]	+	–	–	–	–
CD79a[b]	+	–	–	–	–
CD7, CD2	–	+	±	±	±
Cytoplasmic CD3[a,b]	–	+	–	–	–
CD13[a]	–	–	+	–	±
CD33[a]	–	–	+	+	+
CD117	–	–	±	±	±
omega-MPO[b]	–	–	+	–	–
CD41a/CD61	–	–	–	+	–
Glycophorin A	±	–	–	–	+

[a] sensitive; [b] specific.

+, present; ±, sometimes present; –, absent.

Table 1.4 Common cytogenetic changes in AML in children	
Abnormalities[a]	Approximate proportion positive (%)
+8	14
t(8;21)	12
t(15;17)	9
11q2,3	8
+21	7
inv 16	5
–7	4
del(9q)	4
abn(3q)	2
del(7q)	2
del(5q)	1
–5	1
+22	1

[a] Number in parentheses is the chromosome number.

Table 1.5 Cytogenetic changes in ALL in children	
Abnormalities[a]	Approximate proportion positive (%)
t(12;21)	30
t/del(9)p	8
t/del(12)p	7
del(6)(q)	6
t/del(11)(q)	6
t/del(11)(q) excl.	4
t(1;19)	4
t(4;11)	3
t(9;22)	2
Near haploid (24–29)	1
Hypodiploid (30–45)	9
Pseudodiploid (46)	29
Low hyperdiploid (47–49)	16
High hyperdiploid (50–59)	40
Near triploid (69)	4
Near tetraploid (96)	1

[a] Number in parentheses is the chromosome number.

However, we are gradually moving towards risk-directed therapy and this is already the situation for AML, where low-risk patients are defined as having Inv(16), t(15;17) or t(8;21), whereas high-risk patients have more than five abnormalities or abnormalities of chromosome 5, 7 or 3q (Table 1.6). In infant ALL, the 11q2,3(MLL) gene rearrangement is the most important risk factor. In childhood ALL, abnormalities of 11q are also an indicator of very high-risk, along

Table 1.6 Important risk factors in AML cases	
Prognosis	Risk factors
Poor prognosis: 'high-risk'	−5
	del(5q)
	−7
	abn(3q)
	Failure to remit after first chemotherapy course
	Complex cytogenetic changes (a clone with at least five unrelated cytogenetic changes)
	Secondary AML
Good prognosis: 'low-risk'	t(8;21)
	t(15;17)
	inv(16)
	Down's megakaryoblastic leukaemia (M7)

Table 1.7 Important risk factors in ALL cases	
Prognosis	Risk factors
Poor prognosis: 'high-risk'	MLL gene rearranged in infants
	11q abnormalities
	Philadelphia chromosome (maybe except high hyperdiploid)
	Near haploid chromosome number
	Older age and less than 6 months
	High WBC
	Male gender
	Failure to remit within a month
Good prognosis: 'low-risk'	t (1;19)
	High hyperdiploid
	Age 2–5 years
	Female gender
	Low WBC

with the Philadelphia chromosome t(9;22) (Table 1.7). In myelodysplasias, the presence of chromosome abnormalities similar to those seen with AML (especially monosomy 7) often clinches the diagnosis.

Conclusion

The message of this chapter is a very simple one. The diagnosis of leukaemia is mainly straightforward and can be obvious after taking the history, clinical examination, checking the blood count and film and looking at the bone marrow. However, this can only be reliably carried out by someone who is used to looking at children's bone marrows, and mistakes continue to be made with diagnosis (Table 1.8). The new technologies are of value in terms of prognosis and for the identification of abnormalities, which we hope will be useful in monitoring minimal residual disease. However, it is essential to ensure that all of the results add up to a secure diagnosis and classification in every case and not to act upon anything that does not make sense in comparison with other tests (Box 1.3).

Box 1.3 Important points in the diagnosis of leukaemia

The crucial diagnostic test is bone marrow morphology with MGG or equivalent stain. Other tests are contributory or confirmatory.

The worst mistakes are made when test results are taken in isolation. Nobody should treat leukaemia without having seen the bone marrow slides.

When in doubt, be sure to rule out infections, autoimmune disease and neuroblastoma.

CD13 ± CD33 positivity is common in pre-B ALL. Diagnosis of AML or biphenotypic leukaemia is not justified unless morphology, cytochemistry and rest of immunophenotyping supports this diagnosis.

Diagnosis of true biphenotypic leukaemia can be very difficult and must show myeloid and lymphoid antigens on separate cells.

Beware transient leukaemoid reactions in young babies.

Beware severe aplasia recovering rapidly, it usually prestages leukaemia.

Table 1.8 Mistakes that continue to be made with diagnosis	
Potential error	Examples
Over-reliance on immunophenotyping	Diamond–Blackfan anaemia, viral infections, autoimmune disorders and congenital neutropenias can produce a lymphocytosis and slight excess of blast cells that can be CD10$^+$
Over-reliance on cytogenetic changes	Low-level clones especially monosomy 7 can disappear or not progress for long periods
Over-interpretation of bone marrow morphology	Morphological changes are subjective and are part of an overall picture, e.g. all patients receiving cytotoxic chemotherapy have myelodysplasia. Some patients with neuroblastoma have marrow 'wipe out' along with other clinical features owing to bone involvement and primary tumour
Failure to diagnose infections	Various infections produce (hepato)splenomegaly, cytopenias and an excess of blast cells, e.g. CMV, EBV, HIV, leishmaniasis
Failures of classification because all features are not taken into account	Immunophenotypes may be aberrantly expressed, e.g. CD13/33 frequently found in common ALL; 11q2,3 abnormalities occur in AML and ALL
Aplastic presentation of ALL	A rapidly recovering severe aplasia is usually followed by the development of ALL
Transient abnormal myelopoiesis occurs in young infants	Usually but not always Down's syndrome patients: a leukaemoid reaction that usually does not progress to acute leukaemia

Further reading

Chessells, J.M., Swansbury, G.J., Reeves, P., Bailey, C.C. and Richards, S.M. (1997) Cytogenetics and prognosis in childhood lymphoblastic leukaemia: results of MRC UKALL X. *Leukaemia* 99: 93–100.

Hann, I.M., Lake, B.D., Lilleyman, J.S. and Pritchard, J. (1996) *Colour Atlas of Paediatric Haematology*, 3rd edn. Oxford: Oxford University Press.

Hann, I.M., Richards, S., Eden, O.B. and Hill, F.G.H. (1998) Analysis of the immunophenotype of children treated on the MRC UKALL XI Trial. *Leukaemia* 12: 1249–1255.

Lilleyman, J.S., Hann, I.M. and Blanchette, V. (1998) *Pediatric Hematology*, 2nd edn. Edinburgh: Churchill Livingstone.

Nathan, D. and Oski, S. (1997) *Hematology of Infancy and Childhood*, 5th edn. Philadelphia: Saunders.

Russell, N.H. (1997) Biology of acute leukaemia. Leukaemia series. *Lancet* 349; 188–122.

CHAPTER 2

Management of high-risk and relapsed leukaemia and indications for bone marrow transplantation

P.A. Veys

Introduction

The fact that an increasing number of children with leukaemia are now cured is a noteable achievement of combination chemotherapy schedules. Hence 60–80% of children with ALL and 60% with AML remain disease free following recent treatment schedules. However, there is a significant group of children with high-risk and relapsed disease whose long-term survival remains poor with standard chemotherapy, and in whom intensified chemotherapy protocols and/or bone marrow transplantation (BMT) may be considered. For those children considered for BMT, there is now an expanded pool of volunteer unrelated donors (UD), and for the majority of children who do not have a matched sibling donor (approximately 70%), a suitably matched or single locus mismatched UD can now be found. Some of the indications for BMT remain controversial, and as BMT is associated with considerable toxicity and long-term sequelae, the probability of disease cure by the addition of a transplant procedure must outweigh the higher procedural mortality to warrant its use.

Cure of leukaemia by BMT

The original concept of cure by BMT was through dose intensification, allowing rescue from myeloablative doses of chemotherapy and radiotherapy by infusion of autologous or allogeneic bone marrow cells. Cure of leukaemia by this mechanism depends on the number and chemosensitivity of leukaemic cells present at the time of transplant, and the original concept is strongly supported by the lower relapse rates achieved by carrying out BMT when the patient is in 'remission' rather than 'relapse' from their underlying disease. Hence, most indications for BMT in childhood acute leukaemia now carry the prerequisite that the child has achieved remission prior to BMT. While BMT allows for considerable escalation of chemotherapy dosages, there is a fine line between achieving disease eradication and increasing early mortality from regimen-related toxicity.

There are now several lines of evidence to suggest that alloreactive donor cells can exert an important anti-leukaemic action (reviewed by Antin, 1993). One mechanism of this graft-versus-leukaemia (GVL) effect is mediated by cytotoxic T-cells recognizing major and/or minor histocompatibility antigen (HLA) differences on recipient cells; consequently it also involves cells responsible for graft-versus-host disease (GvHD), although other GVL mechanisms may be more leukaemia specific. Consequently, GVL reactions are more pronounced in the presence of GvHD and/or with increasing donor–recipient HLA disparity, e.g. in transplants from UDs. GVL also appears to be disease specific, with the most powerful GVL effect being observed in CML, and the smallest effect in ALL, presumably owing to co-expression or not of target antigens.

Because the GvHD/GVL effect will not occur and reinfusion of residual leukaemic cells may happen, autologous BMT is predictably associated with a low procedural mortality but a high relapse rate. Despite attempts at *in vitro* purging of leukaemic cells or induction of autologous GvHD with cyclosporin A, the outcome remains disappointing and autologous BMT is no longer utilised as a treatment option in the most recent Medical Research Council (MRC) UKALL R2 and MRC AML 12 paediatric protocols.

Problems in assessing response to BMT

Much debate continues over which children should receive BMT. This problem arises because of the paucity of prospective randomised trials. This occurs frequently because the patient groups have not been large enough to enable randomised studies, and because randomisation, often at the end-stage of the child's disease, is complicated by both patient/family and physician preferences. Much of the available data are, therefore, subject to the bias of patient selection, in particular selection of patients who have achieved and maintained a complete remission until the time of BMT and who, therefore, might fall into a better prognostic group. This can be somewhat offset by censoring patients from 'intent to transplant' or by comparing the outcome of those 'with and without donors' from the outset.

Further problems arise because favourable results of a treatment are more likely to be reported than unfavourable results, giving the impression of greater success from BMT than may be warranted. Conversely, any comparison of the outcome of BMT with chemotherapy requires a prolonged follow-up, because of late leukaemia relapses following chemotherapy.

Which children need BMT?

High-risk ALL in first complete remission

Children with ALL at high risk of relapse may be considered for intensified chemotherapy with or without BMT. Although recent reports suggest that US CCG/POG chemotherapy protocols may be achieving a superior leukaemia-free survival compared with current MRC UKALL schedules, there is little to choose between the various intensified protocols being utilised for the worst risk patients. Those children with

high-risk disease who are currently considered for BMT within the UK are listed in Table 2.1 and account for less than 10% of children with ALL. These children receive intensified chemotherapy with an induction block followed by three consecutive blocks of intensification (except infants who are treated as per infant protocol) before proceeding to BMT. At the present time, a distinction is made between candidates who have a matched family donor (usually sibling) (MSD) available and those without an MSD who would require UD BMT. This has been based on previous inferior outcomes of UD BMT caused by increased rates of GvHD and graft rejection. Several recent studies, however, have confirmed a similar outcome with MSD and UD BMT, and this distinction may now be artificial. In theory, UD BMT may have a survival advantage over MSD BMT in certain high-risk leukaemias, because of an enhanced GVL effect. Patients within these high-risk characteristics have an overall leukaemia-free survival (LFS) at five years of 18–40% with intensive chemotherapy. Reports of BMT in similar groups have achieved a LFS of 62–84%, although this is not censored from intent to transplant. With continuing improvement in high-dose chemotherapy, the definitions of high-risk diseases will need constant re-evaluation.

Relapse of ALL

The prognosis for children who suffer a relapse of ALL depends on the site of the relapse and the duration of the first remission. Short first remissions and bone

Table 2.1 High-risk ALL patients in first complete remission who are candidates for BMT in the UK[a]	
BMT type	Risk factors
For MSD or UD if no sibling available	Philadelphia positive t(9,22)
	Near haploid
For MSD[b]	Failure to remit by day 28 of therapy
	High hazard score
	True biphenotypic leukaemia defined by morphology, markers, cytogenetics

[a] Recommendations by UKCCSG BMT group (1998).

[b] Certain patients may be considered for UD BMT.

marrow relapse carry a worse prognosis, with less than 20% of children with early bone marrow relapse achieving disease eradication even after very intensive salvage therapy. Other factors associated with an adverse prognosis include T-ALL phenotype and circulating blast cells. Children who relapse after a remission of 4 years or more have a high likelihood of achieving a second sustained complete remission (Fig. 2.1). Molecular genetics may also influence prognosis, and the presence of the TEL–AML fusion transcript in relapsed patients may also predict a longer second remission.

Bone marrow relapse

Bone marrow relapse with or without extramedullary relapse of ALL is the most frequent indication for allogeneic BMT in childhood leukaemia. A second remission can normally be achieved in over 80% of children using prednisolone, vincristine, L-asparaginase and an anthracycline, if not restricted by cardiotoxicity. Following reinduction, a number of groups have reported improved survival for children receiving an MSD BMT compared with those who received chemotherapy alone. The probability of leukaemia-free survival following BMT reported in seven comparative studies ranged from 33 to 56% (mean 45%) compared with 9 to 41% (mean 23%) for chemotherapy, with the least benefit in children with long first remissions. Within Europe, MSD BMT is currently regarded as a 'routine' procedure for bone marrow relapse of ALL by the Accreditation Sub-

Committee of the European Group for Blood and Marrow Transplantation (EBMT) (Schmitz *et al.*, 1996). Since the 1990s, children with early relapse of ALL and without an MSD have undergone UD BMT. Overall survival has been significantly better than that reported for adults and a leukaemia-free survival of between 40 and 56% is similar to that with MSD BMT. T-cell depletion methods have reduced the incidence of transplant-related complications, particularly GvHD (100 day mortality 10–20%), and permitted the use of both matched and partially mismatched unrelated donors, so extending the possibility of BMT to most children. Even amongst high-risk patients relapsing on or shortly after stopping therapy, T-cell-depleted UD BMT had a lower relapse rate than that seen for MSD BMT. Between 1985 and 1990, 1612 children with ALL were reported to the UK MRC UKALL X trial: 464 patients who relapsed before the end of October 1993 have been analysed from time of relapse. Of these, 107 children selectively received an allogeneic BMT (81 MSD, 26 UD). Comparison of these with the 297 patients who received salvage chemotherapy alone showed an average reduction in the proportion dying of 11%, from 65% to 54%, corresponding to an odds reduction (OR) of 16% with a standard deviation of 14 ($2P > 0.1$). A similar reduction was seen when selection bias was eliminated by a comparison in outcome between those with and without a donor. The less significant benefits for BMT detailed by this study in comparison with the previous reports reflect the improved survival from the intensified chemotherapy arm; however because of the short follow-up time of the study, further late post-chemotherapy relapses are expected. From the MRC data, the outcome in the group with bone marrow relapse on treatment was significantly better for those treated with BMT than for those treated with chemotherapy alone. There is uniform agreement that children who relapse early have a poor prognosis. Within a group of children with ALL treated at Great Ormond Street Hospital for Children, London, who relapsed within 30 months from diagnosis, none of the 43 patients receiving chemotherapy and only two of the nine receiving MSD BMT became long-term survivors; unfortunately, recent unpublished data from the UKCCSG BMT database suggest that the outcome of UD BMT in children

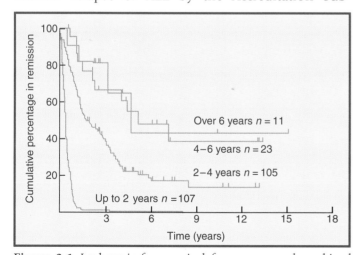

Figure 2.1 *Leukaemia-free survival for marrow and combined relapses according to the length of first complete remission, in children referred to Great Ormond Street Hospital for Children, London, 1972–1990.*

relapsing under 30 months from diagnosis is similarly poor (Fig. 2.2) but is still superior to chemotherapy.

Further reports are awaited to confirm that closely matched UD BMT is an adequate substitute for MSD BMT in children with relapsed ALL. This finding and recent improvements in chemoradiotherapy schedules, which have reduced the relative improvement in benefits of BMT in terms of overall survival, particularly in children with a long first remission, have led to new recommendations for the use of BMT or chemotherapy schedules in children with relapsed ALL (Table 2.2). If a further relapse occurs after salvage chemotherapy and patients achieved a third complete remission, as long as there is not significant organ dysfunction at that stage, then UD BMT should be considered in all patients.

Extramedullary relapse

The management of the small number of children with isolated extramedullary relapse of ALL is more complex. Following CNS relapse, two factors in addition to the length of the first complete remission are important in determining subsequent treatment. These are previous CNS radiotherapy and the presence of a high hazard score, both of which adversely affect the prognosis, increasing the likelihood of a further CNS relapse or subsequent bone marrow relapse,

respectively. Extramedullary relapse off therapy has a better prognosis than bone marrow relapse, and isolated testicular relapse can be cured by chemoradiotherapy alone in 75% of patients. Relapse in the ovaries is rare, usually presenting with an abdominal mass within the first 3 years. Some patients are surviving after intensive retreatment, but there are too few patients to be able to make specific treatment recommendations in this group. Ocular relapses present with local iritis usually within the first year off treatment. Disease control can be achieved with local radiation and intensive chemotherapy, but there is a high risk of subsequent marrow relapse. Recommendations for the treatment of the more common forms of extramedullary relapse of ALL are given in Table 2.2.

New approaches not involving BMT

A number of novel drug combinations have been examined in refractory or second relapse of ALL. Methotrexate and tenoposide, idarubicin and cytarabine, idarubicin with fludarabine and cytarabine, and PEG-L-asparaginase have all shown some activity in this area but none have given lasting benefit. Unfortunately, the newer anthracyclines, *in vitro* at least, have demonstrated significant cross-resistance between the various drugs, and early studies of multidrug resistance and its modulation have not demonstrated any effect of resistance modifiers *in vitro*.

First complete remission in AML

One of the largest studies of paediatric AML, MRC AML 10, accrued 359 children between 1988 and 1995. Prior to AML 10, it was assumed that all children would benefit from an allogeneic BMT if an MSD was available. This was confirmed by a recent multicentre study by the Children's Cancer Group that compared BMT with chemotherapy; this showed a moderate survival advantage for patients eligible for transplantation versus those without a sibling donor, significant at 3 years (53% versus 41%), 5 years (50% versus 36%) and at 8 years (47% versus 34%). The results from AML 10 dispute the concept that all children with AML are candidates for BMT and emphasise the constant requirement to reappraise the need for BMT in the face of improving chemotherapy. It is clear from AML 10 that more intensive

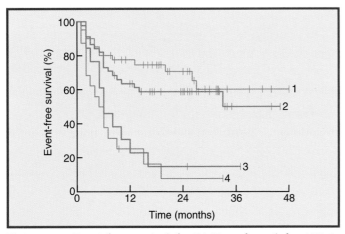

Figure 2.2 *Event-free survival for BMT performed for ALL in second complete remission: 1 = matched sibling donor (MSD), > 24 months from diagnosis to relapse; 2 = unrelated donor (UD), > 24 months from diagnosis to relapse; 3 = UD, ≤ 24 months from diagnosis to relapse; 4 = MSD, ≤ 24 months diagnosis to relapse. The 2-year event-free survival for MSD and UD respectively = 61%, 51% for > 24 months and 8%, 15% for relapse ≤ 24 months (p = 0.00001). (Data taken from the UKCCSG BMT registry March 1998.)*

Table 2.2 Management of relapsed ALL according to duration of first complete remission and site of relapse (MRC Childhood Leukaemia Working Party and UKCCSG BMT group)[a]

Relapse site	Duration of first complete remission		
	< 2.5 years	2.5–4 years	> 4 years
Bone marrow	**UD BMT**[b]	**MSD BMT**	**MSD BMT**
+/- other site	**MSD BMT**[b]	UD BMT or R2 chemotherapy	R2 chemotherapy
Testis	**MSD BMT**	R2 chemotherapy + RT	R2 chemotherapy + RT
	UD BMT or R2 chemotherapy + RT post high-dose methotrexate		
CNS			
Previous CNS RT	**MSD BMT**	**MSD BMT**	R2 chemotherapy + high-dose methotrexate
	UD BMT	UD BMT or R2 chemotherapy + RT	
No previous CNS RT but a high hazard score	**MSD BMT**	R2 chemotherapy + RT	R2 chemotherapy + RT
	UD BMT or R2 chemotherapy + RT		
No previous CNS RT and not a high hazard score	R2 chemotherapy + RT + additional intrathecal methotrexate	R2 chemotherapy + RT	R2 chemotherapy + RT

[a] Preferred options in bold.
[b] Standard practice has been to use an MSD if available; however the results are poor; UD BMT may have a superior GVL effect and is being used in preference in certain cases. R2 chemotherapy, MRC UKALL R2 protocol; RT, radiotherapy to site of relapse. During BMT, testicular or CNS boosts may be given at discretion of clinician.

chemotherapy has improved disease-free survival to 56% at 7 years, with substantially lower relapse rates than both its predecessor AML 9 and the CCG study mentioned above. AML 10 showed that children with favourable karyotype, i.e. t(8;21), t(15;17) and inv(16) had a 7-year survival from complete remission of 78%, regardless of whether they received BMT or not. While not certain, it is likely that 5-year survival equates with cure, as most relapses have occurred in the first 2 years following chemotherapy. Therefore, in the following trial, MRC AML 12, these patients will not receive BMT in first complete remission since the toxicity of the procedure is likely to outweigh any benefit. Higher-risk patients which include children with resistant disease after course 1 (unless they have a favourable karyotype) and all other patients had a survival rate, respectively, of 33% and 61%. Relapse remains the main cause of treatment failure in higher-risk patients, and although MSD BMT did not produce a significant survival benefit, it was considered appropriate to

pursue it because of a lower relapse rate. There still appears to be a 'centre' effect on toxic mortality rates post-BMT and the benefit of BMT may become apparent when supportive care and control of GvHD become widespread.

The role of autologous BMT (ABMT) in first remission ALL also remains uncertain. Most studies include both adults and children and have produced broadly similar results. Probability of disease-free survival is 35–45%, with a risk of leukaemia relapse of 40–60%, and a moderately low death rate due to toxicity of 5–10%. Analysis of the ABMT and chemotherapy-only arms of AML 10 has shown a reduction in relapse following ABMT but no survival difference at 5 years. This is not because of any counter-balancing effect of procedural mortality after ABMT, since there was none. Rather it appears to be related to inferior survival from relapse after ABMT. Three other randomised studies have also not shown any survival benefit of ABMT; therefore, given the substantial long-term morbidity of the procedure, ABMT has been dropped from the AML 12 paediatric protocol altogether.

Second complete remission in AML

The prognosis following relapse of AML is again dependent on the time to relapse. If relapse occurs within 1 year from diagnosis then the outlook is extremely poor. Children relapsing after longer periods may be salvaged with further intensive chemotherapy with or without BMT if they achieve a remission. For children who have not undergone BMT and do not have a sibling donor, re-induction (avoiding cardiotoxic agents), for example with FLAG (fludarabine, cytarabine, granulocyte colony-stimulating factor), followed by ABMT (if late relapse) or UD BMT (if early relapse) in second complete remission are worthwhile approaches.

The overall strategy for the treatment of childhood AML is summarised in Tables 2.3 and 2.4.

Improvements in BMT for acute leukaemia

Leukaemic relapse still remains the most significant problem following BMT in acute leukaemia. There is, therefore, a need for more effective anti-leukaemic regimens and/or enhancement of a GVL effect.

The majority of children undergoing BMT have received cyclophosphamide (Cy) and total body irradiation (TBI) as myeloablative therapy, and although a number of other strategies have been employed, most studies, unfortunately, have been non-comparative. In ALL, several teams have substituted high-dose cytarabine for cyclophosphamide in conjunction with fractionated TBI (ARAC/TBI). The best results were reported from Case Western Reserve Hospital, where 20 paediatric patients had transplants, 58% of whom were alive in continued complete remission, with a relapse rate under 20%. Memorial Sloane Kettering have reported encouraging data from reversing the order of cyclophosphamide/TBI to TBI/cyclophosphamide, with a disease-free survival of children receiving transplants in second complete remission of 64%. From the adult literature, the City of Hope group substituted etoposide (VP16) for cyclophosphamide, and in two studies etoposide/TBI appears to have significant anti-leukaemic activity in refractory ALL. Other investigators, however, have observed considerable toxicity with this regimen, with no improvement in disease-free survival. In an attempt to reduce long-term side effects, other groups have utilised busulphan (Bu) in place of TBI in busulphan/cyclophosphamide. The results were not superior to cyclophosphamide/TBI; however, the studies did illustrate that TBI is not an absolute

Table 2.3 Indications for transplant procedures in childhood AML (adapted from *Proposed Indicators for Transplant Procedures in Children 1997*, developed through the UKCCSG BMT group)

Disease status	Allogeneic matched related	Allogeneic unrelated	Autologous blood or marrow
CR1	R[a]	NR	NR
CR2	R	CRP[b]	R[b]
Relapse/refractory	D	D	NR

CR1, first complete remission; CR2, second complete remission; R, in routine use for selected patients; CRP, to be undertaken in approved Clinical Research Protocols; D, developmental or pilot studies can be approved in specialist units; NR, not generally recommended.

[a] Not t(15;17), t(8;21), inv(16), Down's syndrome.
[b] See Table 2.4.

Table 2.4 Management of relapsed AML in second complete remission

Previous treatment	Management
No BMT	MSD BMT
	Consider UD BMT if relapse <1 year from diagnosis
	Auto BMT if relapse >1 year from diagnosis (with CR1 marrow)
Autologous BMT	Consider UD BMT if relapse >6 months since auto BMT
MSD BMT	Donor T-cell infusion
	Second MSD BMT if >12 months since first BMT

MSD, matched sibling (or family) donor (including 5/6 HLA matches in certain cases); UD, unrelated donor; CR, complete remission.

requirement for successful treatment of ALL with BMT. However, in a recent large case-matched study from the EBMT registry, patients undergoing ABMT for ALL other than for ALL in first complete remission had a significantly higher probability of relapse with busulphan/cyclophosphamide (84%) than with cyclophosphamide/TBI (62%), translating into a significant difference in 2-year, leukaemia-free survival in favour of cyclophosphamide/TBI (34% versus 13%).

For pre-BMT preparation of patients with AML, the combination of melphalan/TBI may reduce the relapse rate after BMT compared with cyclophosphamide/TBI, but it is associated with increased transplant-related toxicity and no survival advantage. Busulphan/ cyclophosphamide was introduced with a view to reducing transplant-related mortality, but as yet no survival advantage over cyclophosphamide/TBI has been demonstrated, and the results of a recent French collaborative trial have shown that patients prepared with cyclophosphamide/TBI had a significantly better 2-year, disease-free survival than patients prepared with busulphan/cyclophosphamide (72% versus 47%) and a significantly lower relapse rate (14% versus 34%). In the recent case-matched study from the EBMT registry, no significant differences in terms of treatment-related mortality, relapse and leukaemia-free survival for both ABMT and MSD BMT were found between busulphan/cyclophosphamide and cyclophosphamide/TBI. The addition of melphalan to mini busulphan/cyclophosphamide (Bu16/Cy120) has yielded exciting early results in paediatric myelodysplasia.

Children relapsing with leukaemia since the 1990s are likely to have received more intensive chemotherapy prior to transplant, and it is probable that simple intensification of the pre-BMT conditioning alone may not improve leukaemia-free survival in these patients; although incorporation of leukaemia-specific immunotoxins into the pre-transplant regimen may achieve further disease eradication without the added toxicity of conventional therapy. Alternatively, attempts have been made to augment a GVL effect by post-transplant immunotherapy using cytokines, e.g. interleukin 2 or interferon, reduction of GvHD prophylaxis, or infusion of donor T-cells after the transplant. Attempts

have been made to improve disease eradication following ABMT by purging leukaemia cells from the harvested marrow with mafosfamide, monoclonal antibodies or long-term culture. Attempts have also been made to induce autologous GVL with cyclosporin A. Results are awaited from prospective studies to assess whether there is any clinical benefit from any of these manoeuvres.

Myelodysplastic and myeloproliferative syndromes

A recent classification and prognostic scoring system for paediatric myelodysplasia (MDS) has been described (Passmore *et al.*, 1995). The classification has been broadened to include not only those disorders included in the French–American–British (FAB) classification of MDS, but also specific paediatric syndromes including juvenile myelomonocytic leukaemia (JMML) and infantile monosomy 7 syndrome (IMo7). The progression to AML in this large group of paediatric patients was 25%, and the group as a whole responded poorly to intensive chemotherapy or succumbed to infection during prolonged periods of marrow failure. BMT from an MSD, therefore, appears to be the most effective form of treatment for myelodysplasias in childhood; the use of UD BMT is under investigation. The optimum timing, the type of preparative regimen and the role of pre-transplant chemotherapy and/or splenectomy remain to be defined. A recent report from the European Working Group on Myelodysplastic Syndrome in Childhood suggested the use of an MSD as opposed to alternative donors, the use of chemotherapy as opposed to TBI in the preparative regimen, and promoting GVL via the use of mild rather than intensive GvHD prophylaxis, all lead to an improved event-free survival. Recommendations for the treatment of childhood MDS are shown in Figure 2.3.

Classical Philadelphia chromosome-positive CML is rare in childhood, and, as in adults, the only curative therapy is ABMT. If an MSD is not available, then a matched UD should be sought, with the best results being obtained from BMT within the first year of the chronic phase of the disease. Results are much poorer in the advanced phase of the disease and following blast crisis.

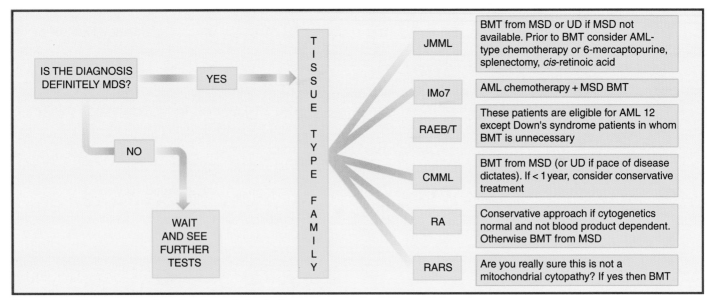

Figure 2.3 *Management of paediatric myelodysplasia.*

In the adult setting, CML has been shown to be particularly susceptible to a GVL effect, with an increased incidence of relapse following T-cell-depleted BMT and induction of subsequent remissions with donor leucocyte transfusions.

Treatment of relapse following transplantation

Relapse after an uncomplicated BMT presents a difficult problem. Parents frequently wish to pursue further attempts at cure. The toxicity of a second BMT is considerable, and leukaemia-free survival is very poor: <10% if the relapse is within 6 months of the first BMT. For later relapses, leukaemia-free survival may be better, and second BMT should not be considered unless relapse occurs at least 1 year after initial BMT. If a second BMT is undertaken, attempts should be made to increase GVL activity by using a T-replete graft and/or reducing GvHD prophylaxis. In relapse of adult CML following T-cell-depleted BMT, infusion of donor T lymphocytes (DLI) may achieve a further remission without further preparative treatment, although induction of severe GvHD and marrow aplasia may be problematic. The benefits of such procedures following relapse of childhood acute leukaemia after BMT, particularly when the initial graft is T-cell replete, remain unknown. The current approach in children involves re-inducing remission with vincristine/prednisolone/asparaginase in ALL and a high-dose cytosine-containing regimen (e.g. FLAG) in AML and proceeding to DLI, with incremental doses of T-cells (10^6–10^8 cells/kg) depending on donor compatibility at intervals of 4–8 weeks. Such procedures are additionally complicated by practical and ethical issues over re-use of child donors. Alpha-interferon has also been utilised both before DLI in relapsed CML and after DLI in relapsed acute leukaemia to induce GVL.

Further reading

Antin, J.H. (1993) Graft-versus-leukaemia: no longer an epiphenomenon, *Blood* 82: 2273–2277.

Passmore, S.J., Hann, I.M., Stiller, C.A. *et al.* (1995) Paediatric myelodysplasia: a study of 68 children and a new prognostic scoring system. *Blood* 85: 1742–1750.

Schmitz, N., Gratwohl, A. and Goldman, J.M. (1996) Allogeneic and autologous transplantation for haematological diseases, tumours and immune disorders. Current practice in Europe in 1996 and proposals for an operational classification. *Bone Marrow Transplant* 17: 471–477.

CHAPTER 3

Complications of therapy for haematological malignancies

N. Goulden, P.A. Veys and D.K.H. Webb

Introduction

Cure rates for acute leukaemias and lymphomas have improved since the 1980s, primarily because of increased intensity of chemotherapy. This has occurred at the cost of greater toxicity, and the most intensive regimens (for example for AML and mature B-cell lymphoma/leukaemia) carry high rates of morbidity and mortality: in the UK around 10% of children with AML or advanced B-cell lymphoma have died through treatment-related complications. The toxic death rate for ALL and T-cell non-Hodgkin's lymphoma (T-NHL) is lower at 2–5% in line with the lower intensity of therapy. Deaths occur primarily because of infection, with bleeding, metabolic disturbances (including tumour lysis syndrome), and second tumours as the remaining leading causes of death following chemotherapy (Table 3.1). For those children receiving a bone marrow transplant, GvHD is a major cause of death.

A wide range of complications is recognised that are not usually fatal but are the cause of considerable morbidity. New aspects of this morbidity continue to be recognised, with anthracycline-related cardiac toxicity and venous thrombosis particular examples of previously under-recognised complications. With the generally high survival rates for childhood leukaemias and lymphomas, better understanding of mechanisms and the possible benefits of treatment modifications (e.g. reduced levels of anthracyclines) and preventative strategies (e.g. the use of cardioprotectants) are fundamental.

Table 3.1 Causes of death in children treated for ALL and AML in the MRC UKALL X and AML 10 trials

Cause of death	ALL[a]	AML[b]
Infection	68	28
bacteria	33	9
fungal	16	7
viral	16	1
Pneumocystis carinii	3	0
Bleeding	4	10
Metabolic disorders	3	0
Cardiac toxicity	0	9[c]
Second tumour	13	2
Other	3	4

[a] $n = 91$ (from Wheeler *et al.*, 1996).

[b] $n = 47$ (from L. Riley, personal communication).

[c] Eight children developed cardiac failure in association with sepsis.

Hyperleucocytosis

A white cell count in excess of 100×10^9 cells/l occurs in 10% of children with acute leukaemia and is generally accompanied by anaemia, which compensates blood viscosity. Symptoms of hyperviscosity are uncommon even in children with very high counts. Simple 'top-up' transfusion is contraindicated prior to cytoreduction, to avoid raising blood viscosity further. Children usually tolerate even severe anaemia well and transfusion can be deferred until the white cell count has fallen in the majority of patients; the early institution of cytoreductive chemotherapy is effective and leucapheresis or exchange transfusion in small children is rarely required. In children with heart failure or very extreme anaemia exchange transfusion or leucapheresis can be used partially to correct both white cell count and anaemia but should be accompanied by cytoreductive chemotherapy as otherwise the white cell count shows rapid rebound. It is generally possible to hyperhydrate and treat with allopurinol for several hours prior to therapy to reduce the likelihood of tumour lysis syndrome.

Platelet support

The approach to platelet support has varied and although the only absolute indication for transfusion is bleeding or the need to cover an invasive procedure, arbitrary thresholds for platelet transfusion have often been set at around 20×10^9 cells/l in otherwise well children, with a higher threshold in the presence of sepsis or abnormal coagulation screens. In the absence of sepsis or bleeding, very low levels ($5–10 \times 10^9$) are often tolerated and there is no indication to give platelets because of petechiae or bruises only. It remains appropriate to maintain a higher platelet count ($>50 \times 10^9$ cells/l) in patients with sepsis or DIC. Most children do not develop refractoriness to platelet transfusions, but HLA-matched donations are useful in children with demonstrated anti-HLA antibodies.

Neutropenia

Reductions in the severity, frequency and duration of neutropenia are a major goal of supportive care, but the use of granulocyte or granulocyte–macrophage colony-stimulating factors (G-CSF or GM-CSF) has not generally been beneficial as these drugs do not abrogate the initial phase of neutropenia but rather shorten the total duration. Accordingly, treated children still tend to develop febrile neutropenia and to require hospital admission for supportive care. Recommendations regarding the use of growth factors are summarised in Box 3.1. In a similar fashion, it remains unlikely that thrombopoietin will have a major impact following chemotherapy.

Box 3.1 Indications for the use of G-CSF in haematological malignancies

To accelerate neutrophil recovery after BMT

To mobilise stem cells for peripheral blood stem cell collections

To accelerate neutrophil recovery in children with proven unresponsive bacterial or fungal infection despite appropriate antimicrobial therapy. (GM-CSF may be more appropriate for fungal infection.)

Patterns of infection

Patterns of infection change and in the 1990s Gram-positive organisms have emerged as the most commonly isolated bacteria (Table 3.2). One factor may be the widespread adoption of long-term central venous catheters for treatment delivery and supportive care, but the reasons for this change are ill-defined. However, as deaths are generally associated with the minority of documented infections caused by Gram-negative organisms, initial selection of antibiotics remains focussed on adequate therapy for these bacteria, with a general recommendation of double Gram-negative cover (usually a β-lactam antibiotic and an aminoglycoside) as initial therapy for febrile neutropenia.

The use of prophylactic antibiotics, gut decontamination or the routine prescription of haemopoietic

Table 3.2 Organisms isolated in children with febrile neutropenia

Type of infection	Incidence (%)
Proven bacterial	27
Gram positive	17
Gram negative	8
Polymicrobial	2
Proven fungal	6
Proven viral	14
Mixed	1
Pyrexia of unknown origin	49
Non-infective	3

From Hann et al. (1997).

growth factors (G-CSF or GM-CSF) during periods of neutropenia do not bestow a clear benefit and are not indicated for the majority of children.

The policy of early initiation of antibiotics for febrile neutropenia (usually defined as fever above 38°C for 4 hours or a single episode of 39°C with neutrophils <0.5 × 10^9 cells/l) has reduced deaths caused by Gram-negative septicaemia, but this improvement has been complicated by the emergence of opportunist infection by fungi (mainly *Candida* and *Aspergillus* spp.) and, to a lesser extent, viruses.

Meningitis is extremely unusual as a cause of febrile neutropenia and, accordingly, a lumbar puncture does not form a routine part of the assessment; initial chest radiographs in children without respiratory symptoms or signs do not generally lead to a change in antibiotics.

Clinical examination must be thorough and include observation of the perineum to exclude cellulitis.

Fungal infections

Prolonged neutropenia and the use of broad-spectrum antibiotics are risk factors for fungal sepsis, and, accordingly, proven infection is most common in children receiving highly intensive chemotherapy. Bacterial cultures are positive in less than half of the patients and persistence of fever beyond 96 hours with negative cultures indicates the need for empiric antifungal therapy (Fig. 3.1) with amphotericin (the spectrum of fluconazole is insufficient in this setting, and the role of itraconazole is unproven), although this agent results in significant toxicity with febrile reactions (45% of patients), rigors (50%), renal impairment (34%) and hypokalaemia owing to renal tubular losses. There are clear advantages to the use of liposomal amphotericin in its reduced toxicity and ease of administration, but the use of this agent is often restricted because of its high cost. Indications for the cost-effective use of this drug are given in Box 3.2. Amphotericin B is adequate and reasonably tolerated in most children as empirical therapy, with liposomal preparations reserved for those with proven fungal infection or intolerable side effects, including severe hypokalaemia despite replacement and potassium-sparing diuretics, renal impairment or severe allergic reactions.

Investigation of persistent fever should include a chest radiograph, an echocardiogram for children with

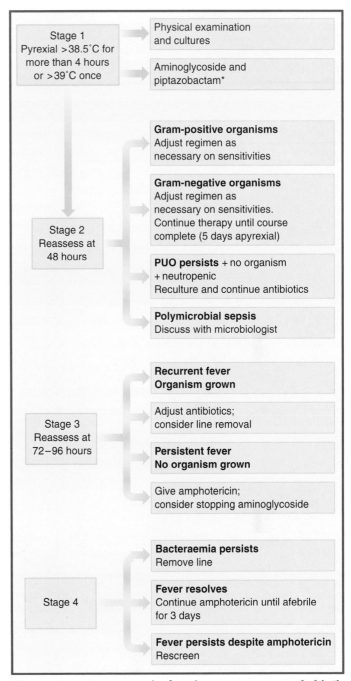

Figure 3.1 *An approach for the management of febrile neutropenia in children. *If intravenous piptazobactam has been previously given, use ceftazidime plus an aminoglycoside. If ceftazidime has been used in the previous 2 weeks, or ceftazidime-resistant organisms are involved/suspected, use ciprofloxacin plus an aminoglycoside first.*

a central venous line, imaging (preferably CT scan) of the abdomen for fungal microabcesses of liver or spleen, which may only become visible following neutrophil recovery, and radiographs of the paranasal sinuses as a potential site of aspergillosis. Areas of consolidation on a chest radiograph should be treated

> **Box 3.2 Indications for liposomal amphotericin in febrile neutropenia**
>
> Proven fungal infection inadequately responsive to standard amphotericin
>
> Persistent fever and negative cultures for 96 hours despite appropriate broad-spectrum antibiotics plus at least one of the following:
>
> - impaired renal function (creatinine more than twice normal)
> - impaired liver function (transaminases more than three times normal)
> - severe hypokalaemia (<2.5 mmol/l) despite potassium-sparing diuretic and replacement therapy
> - BMT patient taking cyclosporin
> - severe reactions to standard amphotericin despite premedication with steroid, antihistamine or pethidine

with circumspection, and a CT scan may demonstrate features of *Aspergillus* infection, indicating a need for bronchoscopy, bronchoalveolar lavage and possible surgery.

Central-line infections

In children with infections associated with long-term central venous catheters, it is possible to clear infection in the majority of these patients with adequate (10 days) and appropriate intravenous antibiotics, remembering to alternate lumens for antibiotic administration in children with double lumen catheters. In many cases, the organism will be a coagulase-negative staphylococcus, many of which are resistant to most routine anti-microbials other than vancomycin and teicoplanin. Either of these agents is suitable therapy: teicoplanin has the advantage of single daily dosing after the first day of treatment, which is especially useful for outpatient therapy. For children with recurrent or persistent infection despite adequate courses of treatment, line removal is advisable. Tunnel infections involving the line track usually require line removal, although exit site sepsis, when present, is often chronic and low grade or recurrent during neutropenic episodes and is usually easier to control.

Viral infections

The most problematic viral infections are chicken pox and measles, and appropriate immunoglobulin prophylaxis is mandatory for all non-immune children who are direct contacts with infectious cases (Box 3.3). Established chicken pox requires therapy with high-dose intravenous aciclovir for at least 10 days, but there remains no satisfactory therapy for measles infection. Although cytomegalovirus (CMV) infection is of major importance following BMT, it is an uncommon cause of serious morbidity after standard chemotherapy, although acute infection may produce infectious mononucleosis and, very rarely, pneumonitis. Parvovirus B19 infection in immunocompromised children produces prolonged erythroid hypoplasia that responds to intravenous immunoglobulin, and this should be excluded in children with recurrent or persistent marked anaemia by serology. The prevalence of hepatitis C infection shows geographical variation and has been documented in 1–16% of children treated for leukaemia/lymphoma, with a higher incidence in more heavily transfused children, particularly those receiving BMT. Infected children are eligible for and should be enrolled in clinical trials of alpha-interferon therapy and should in any case be treated if they have persistently elevated transaminases and biopsy evidence of hepatic fibrosis. Although responses to interferon are affected by viral genotype (type 1 is less responsive), around 30% of patients derive sustained benefit to prolonged courses (12 months or more), and combination therapies, for

> **Box 3.3 Aspects of vaccination and prevention of viral infections in children on chemotherapy**
>
> Children should not receive live vaccines while on therapy, within 6 months from the end of chemotherapy, or for 12 months after BMT. This period may be extended for continued immunosuppressive drugs or complications (e.g. GvHD).
>
> The healthy siblings of children on cancer therapy should only receive inactivated polio vaccine but can and should be given measles–mumps–rubella (MMR) vaccine as necessary. It is not appropriate to separate siblings from children on chemotherapy following MMR vaccination.
>
> All children requiring chemotherapy must have their chicken pox and measles immune status determined. Non-immune children require immunoglobulin prophylaxis as early as possible following a close contact with a child who is infectious for chicken pox or measles. Children should not generally be kept off school because there are children in the community with these infections.

example ribavirin (tribavirin) with interferon, may increase response rates.

Tumour lysis syndrome

Tumour lysis syndrome occurs most commonly in children with high-count ALL or bulky B-cell lymphoma. Renal function may be especially compromised by renal infiltration or obstruction of the outflow tract in children with abdominal and pelvic B-cell NHL, and these children may require initial management with dialysis before treatment can be safely administered; if there is doubt regarding renal function prior to initiation of therapy for B-cell ALL/NHL, it is wise to arrange protective dialysis. Conventional prehydration (3 l/m² daily of 4% dextrose/0.18% NaCl with no added potassium) and allopurinol to prevent urate nephropathy may be inadequate, and alternative agents to control hyperuricaemia, for example uricozyme, may be beneficial. Alkalinisation of the urine is no longer appropriate as a standard precaution. Moderate increases in potassium and phosphate levels may be controlled by further increases in hyperhydration, and asymptomatic hypocalcaemia associated with hyperphosphataemia is usually not corrected. Extremely careful monitoring of fluid balance and electrolytes is essential, with blood sampling and assessment of fluid balance charts at least every 4–6 hours throughout the first few days. Children at high risk, especially those with advanced B-cell NHL, should only be treated in institutions equipped to intervene rapidly with dialysis where necessary.

Disorders of haemostasis

Changes in the levels of platelets and coagulation factors caused by both disease and drugs are well documented at diagnosis and during induction chemotherapy. DIC may occur in any malignancy but is particularly associated with acute promyelocytic (AML FAB type M3) and acute monocytic leukaemia (FAB type M5), because of the procoagulant activity of blast cell cytoplasmic granules and enzymes. AML M3 was associated with a high mortality during the induction phase because of bleeding, despite coagulation factor and platelet replacement and low-dose heparin prophylaxis, but the widespread use of *all-trans*-retinoic acid (ATRA) during induction has largely alleviated this complication. Clinical trials indicate that ATRA should be started at the beginning of induction therapy and continued until complete remission. Some patients develop an 'ATRA syndrome' with fever, weight gain, respiratory distress and pulmonary infiltrates, which can progress to multiorgan failure. The mechanism of this disorder is unknown, although it may result from dysregulation in production of or altered sensitivity to cytokines. The ATRA syndrome can occur at any white cell count, but the risk is increased by high counts (in this context >20 × 10⁹ cells/l). Although remission may be induced by ATRA alone, the contemporaneous use of cytotoxic chemotherapy reduces the risk of the ATRA syndrome, particularly as the use of ATRA may cause a rise in white cell count, and is essential for cure. Dexamethasone is beneficial for patients with evidence of the ATRA syndrome, whereas cytoreduction by leucapheresis seems ineffective.

Thrombotic disease

The prevalence of thrombotic disease has increased during the 1990s with estimates of 1–15% from different studies of children given ALL therapy. Partly this increase in prevalence figures is caused by increased awareness and more comprehensive assessments, particularly the use of Doppler ultrasound, lineograms and venograms to assess line and vessel patency in children with long-term central venous lines. Contributory factors include hyperleucocytosis, asparaginase therapy and central venous catheters. CNS thrombosis is the most commonly reported site (Table 3.3), probably reflecting the severity of this complication, but clots associated with venous catheters are probably under-recorded, although this suggests that many of these episodes do not carry immediate clinical significance. Many children have evidence of thrombosis of vessels containing central lines when venography has been undertaken, even when the line itself remains patent; intermittent episodes of line blockage may represent thrombosis at the catheter tip. The appropriate

Table 3.3 Sites of thrombosis in children treated for acute lymphoblastic leukaemia	
Site	Incidence (% of cases)
Central nervous system	65
Deep veins	16
Pulmonary embolus	3
Combinations	7
Site unknown	10
From Mitchell, Sutor and Andrew (1995).	

management of these episodes is contentious, and the role of preventative anticoagulation remains unproven. However, episodes of major vessel occlusion or thrombi in the right atrium are generally treated with anticoagulation preceded or accompanied by fibrinolysis with recombinant tissue plasminogen activator (r-tPA) or surgical removal of the clot from the atrium. The use of continued or preventative anticoagulation produces difficulties in planning invasive procedures, for example, lumbar punctures for intrathecal prophylaxis, if warfarin is used, but low-molecular-weight heparin can be discontinued temporarily to allow these procedures, despite the disadvantage of administration by regular subcutaneous injections. The need for therapy with less significant catheter-associated thrombosis is controversial and requires formal randomised studies. One justification for intervention is the risk of long-term morbidity owing to the post-thrombotic syndrome, although this complication has not been described in our follow-up clinic despite a conservative policy for the investigation and management of catheter-related problems. This issue needs adequate prospective studies to determine optimal management, as registry data are likely to show reporting biases.

Neuropathy and myopathy

Neurological complications occur in around 10% of children and include peripheral neuropathies, most commonly associated with vincristine, and myopathies (steroid related). Loss of ankle jerks is common with vincristine, but more severe weakness such as foot

drop, severe constipation and bone pain require temporary cessation of therapy pending recovery, and re-introduction of vincristine at reduced dosage. Involvement of the recurrent laryngeal nerve(s) is uncommon but results in vocal cord paresis, hoarseness and possible breathing/swallowing difficulties. This complication has occurred early in therapy and the possible role of vincristine should be remembered in children who develop vocal cord paresis but who may also have received surgical procedures to the neck or mediastinum.

Seizures

Seizures occur in up to 10% of children receiving treatment for ALL and are associated with the induction, CNS prophylaxis and intensification phases of treatment rather than continuation therapy; seizures are rarely, if ever, a manifestation of CNS relapse. Causes of seizures include CNS thrombosis and haemorrhage, metabolic disturbances, infections and drugs, particularly methotrexate (both parenteral and intrathecal), asparaginase and vincristine. Investigations should include plasma chemistry and CNS imaging, but the prognosis is generally good and recurrence is unusual in the absence of structural changes or preceding neurological deficit/dysfunction. In most cases of drug-related seizures, further methotrexate can be administered safely, although further asparaginase is contraindicated if CNS thrombosis has occurred.

Encephalopathies are well described in children treated for leukaemia and lymphoma and are caused by metabolic alterations, disorders of haemostasis and thrombosis, drug toxicities and viral and fungal infections. Appropriate investigation includes a blood count, biochemical assessment, a coagulation screen, CNS imaging, and microbiology. Implicated viruses include herpes simplex, chicken pox, measles and mumps; amongst fungi, Candida, Aspergillus and Cryptococcus spp. are noteworthy.

Leucoencephalopathy complicates CNS-directed therapy, particularly in children receiving frequent or high-dose intrathecal/intravenous methotrexate following cranial radiation; to avoid this, high-dose methotrexate and cranial radiation should not be given within 12 months of each other. The spectrum of symptoms and signs is variable and includes confusion, coma, tremor, seizures, hemiplegia and dementia; the incidence of the disorder increases with the dose intensity of methotrexate, the combination of methotrexate with radiation, delivery of chemotherapy via intraventricular reservoirs, and a history of CNS leukaemia. Leucoencephalopathy is rare with modern treatment schedules but continues to be reported in the setting of continued intrathecal methotrexate following BMT for relapsed disease.

Cardiac toxicity

Estimates of echocardiographic abnormalities (measurements of left ventricular systolic stress and contractility) in children following treatment for acute leukaemia range from 25 to 65%, depending on treatment protocol and cumulative doses of anthracyclines. It is clear that there is no completely 'safe' dose of these drugs, although cardiac dysfunction and arrhythmias consequent on myocardial necrosis and fibrosis are dose related. From 3 to 10% of children receiving cumulative doses of 395 mg/m^2 or more develop cardiac failure within 1 year of completion of anthracyclines, and even if the acute episode is successfully treated, a proportion recur and require heart transplants. In one UK study, 16 children were recorded as having had referral for cardiac transplant following successful treatment for cancer, of whom three were treated for AML. Following exposure to 240–680 mg/m^2 of anthracyclines, the 5-year actuarial survival post-transplant was 75% in this small cohort. Strategies to reduce toxicity include dose restrictions, extended infusions and the use of cardioprotectants. However, adequate randomised trials to assess efficacy and safety are lacking, and so the role of various cardioprotection strategies are inadequately defined. Mediastinal irradiation accentuates anthracycline cardiotoxicity and should be avoided wherever possible. The cumulative exposure to anthracyclines is of particular concern in high-dose schedules, for example in AML therapy, and raises particular issues regarding the choice of regimen following relapse, especially when a BMT with associated exposure to radiotherapy or other cardiotoxins is likely. Accordingly relapsed children with AML in the UK are currently recommended to receive fludarabine, cytarabine and G-CSF (FLAG) as reinduction therapy, and total body irradiation is avoided in preparative regimens for BMT in second remission.

Gastrointestinal toxicity

Mucositis is common following intensive phases of therapy and is an important cause of morbidity. Severe mucositis is associated with very intensive chemotherapy (particularly cytarabine, anthracyclines and alkylating agents) and total body irradiation, for example protocols for AML, B-cell NHL/ALL and following BMT, but it is rarely a cause of death. Severe fluid losses, electrolyte abnormalities and severe pain may result and infants are especially vulnerable to massive diarrhoea, dehydration and disturbed biochemistry. Accordingly, very careful observation with early intervention and aggressive fluid and electrolyte support is mandatory for these high-risk patients. On occasion, there may be peritonism and ileus, raising anxieties of a surgical complication, although these severe cases almost always settle with adequate supportive care and analgesia, and surgical intervention is rarely appropriate. It is very important that these children receive adequate analgesia (this frequently means opiates) at all times.

Hepatic toxicity

Abnormalities in liver function tests are common during chemotherapy because of drug-induced hepatitis, although elevations of transaminases are usually mild and intermittent. Mild periportal inflammatory changes and fatty infiltration are seen on biopsy, although portal fibrosis is less common and associated with prolonged continuation therapy. Very rarely, portal hypertension has developed as a late effect of treatment. Methotrexate, mercaptopurine and asparaginase are all recognised hepatotoxins that are standard drugs in ALL and NHL therapy. Occasionally marked elevations in transaminases occur following treatments but provided there is return to near normal, further treatment may continue. Veno-occlusive disease of the liver has rarely been reported following standard leukaemia chemotherapy and is more typically associated with BMT (see below).

Allogeneic BMT

Complications of allogeneic BMT can be divided into four broad categories: toxicity resulting from the conditioning regimen, infection as a result of immunosuppression, graft failure and GvHD. Collectively, these contribute to a transplant-related mortality of 10–20% in children. In the following section, we have concentrated on two specific issues. These are hepatic veno-occlusive disease, for which new therapies have recently become available, and the management of post-transplant immunodeficiency, which is increasingly important in the era of alternative donor transplants.

Veno-occlusive disease of the liver

Definition

Hepatic veno-occlusive disease (VOD) is a clinical syndrome characterised by painful hepatomegaly, fluid retention and hyperbilirubinaemia that develops within the first month after transplant. It results from injury to the endothelium of hepatic veins and sinusoids and hepatocytes in zone 3 of the liver acinus, which appears to be directly caused by conditioning therapy. Hepatomegaly and weight gain are often detectable at day 0 and hyperbilirubinaemia develops at a median of day +6.

Incidence

It is not possible to give reliable figures for the overall incidence of VOD after paediatric BMT as there is a wide variation in the definition of VOD between centres, but it seems likely that as many as 50% of children receiving a BMT may fulfil the Seattle criteria (Box 3.4) for a diagnosis of VOD. Of 50 allografts performed each year in our centre, 20 are considered to be at high risk of VOD (60 × 3.5). Approximately half of these will develop clinically significant VOD in spite of prophylaxis. In the majority of patients the process will be self limiting and requires no specific

---

Box 3.4 Criteria for the diagnosis of veno-occlusive disease (see Bearman, 1995)

Seattle criteria for VOD (McDonald)

Two of the following three symptoms:
- jaundice (bilirubin >27 mmol/l)
- weight gain >2%
- tender hepatomegaly

Baltimore criteria for VOD (Jones)

Jaundice (bilirubin >34 mmol/l) and any two of the following:
- weight gain >5%
- hepatomegaly
- ascites

Severity of VOD

Severity of VOD is defined retrospectively:
- mild disease spontaneously resolves without specific intervention
- moderate disease requires treatment but resolves before day 100
- severe disease is defined as leading to death or persisting beyond day 100

---

intervention. Fulminant synthetic hepatic failure is uncommon and the major cause of morbidity and mortality is multiorgan failure. In the most severely affected children, renal and cardiopulmonary failure develop within a week of the onset of weight gain.

Diagnosis

Two sets of diagnostic criteria have been published (Box 3.4). Supportive but non-specific findings include renal impairment and refractoriness to platelet transfusion. Microangiopathic haemolysis within the liver may lead to artificially high platelet counts in automated analysers because of the presence of red cell fragments: regular assessment of blood films is, therefore, recommended.

Ultrasound is widely used in the assessment of patients with suspected VOD, although it often serves only to confirm the clinical impression of hepatomegaly and ascites. Gall bladder thickening is a non-specific finding, and reversal of portal venous flow is a late event. Whereas measurements of hepatic artery resistance and colour flow Doppler analyses are abnormal in clinically apparent VOD, these have not been widely validated. Moreover, there is no evidence that they are of predictive value during the early phase of the illness.

Percutaneous liver biopsy is contraindicated in the immediate post-transplant period but transvenous biopsies have been carried out safely in some units. However, this technique is not widely available and may be impractical in smaller children. Studies from Seattle and Barcelona suggest that, while adequate specimens could be obtained by this route, diagnostic biopsies were restricted to patients with clinically obvious VOD and accordingly there is no place for liver biopsy to confirm a diagnosis of VOD within the first month after transplant.

The differential diagnosis of VOD before engraftment is limited and includes drug toxicity, fungal infection, right heart failure, hyperacute GvHD and cholestasis secondary to sepsis. However, the triad of hyperbilirubinaemia, fluid retention and painful hepatomegaly is normally diagnostic. Following engraftment, the diagnosis may be confused by the co-existence of GvHD or viral hepatitis, and at this time more aggressive investigation may be required.

Management

There is currently no proven safe therapy for established VOD; accordingly management involves selection of children deemed to be at high risk for the development of VOD for prophylaxis and providing supportive care for established disease. Although independent risk factors have been identified, there is no substitute for local audit and clinical experience. There is good evidence that patients with antecedent biochemical hepatitis and those receiving T-cell-replete grafts are at higher risk of VOD. It has also become clear that there is significant inter-patient variation in the metabolism of busulphan and that patients with high levels have an increased risk of VOD. It is our practice to measure the area under the curve (AUC) at 7 hours after initial busulphan dose and modify subsequent doses accordingly. Box 3.5 lists the risk factors for the development of VOD after allogeneic BMT.

Conventional definitions of the severity of VOD are based on retrospective assessments (Box 3.4). This approach is of no value to the clinician faced with a decision as to whether to intervene in a child with VOD. Logistic regression models, based on the rate of

> **Box 3.5 Risk factors for the development of VOD after allogeneic BMT**
>
> Busulphan level (AUC at 7 hours) >2,000 mmol/l
>
> Use of melphalan, thiotepa or etoposide in addition to busulphan
>
> Biochemical hepatitis in the 6-month period prior to BMT
>
> Previous cryptosporidial infection in children with combined immunodeficiency

weight gain and increase in bilirubin, have been used to predict outcome, but these require extensive local experience and may not be applicable to all preparative regimens. A more pragmatic (and clinically useful) system is to use a local definition of clinically significant VOD and to this end we institute specific supportive measures in patients who fulfil the Baltimore criteria (Table 3.4).

Supportive measures

The supportive regimen is based on the maintenance of adequate intravascular volume with regular albumin infusions, judicious use of diuretics and sodium restriction, and careful monitoring of girth and fluid balance. Steroids are used if transaminitis develops. It is important to note that the urea will almost inevitably rise in these patients because of their hypercatabolic state and heavy protein load, but the plasma creatinine remains a reliable indicator of renal function in this situation. Adequate analgesia and continued attention to nutrition are mandatory. Paracentesis may be required either for respiratory embarrassment or to relieve discomfort. This procedure may be technically difficult in a sick young child and should only be undertaken in a controlled sterile environment.

Clinically significant VOD resolves with supportive care in the majority of patients. In a minority, rapid progression to multiorgan failure occurs and in a further subset a steady state of ascites and fluid retention may persist for several months. Attempts to alter the natural history of VOD have met with only limited success and it is not possible to recommend any specific measure confidently. This problem is compounded by the fact that it is not possible to predict reliably the clinical course of VOD early in the process.

Table 3.4 Management of hepatic VOD	
Patient group	Management strategy
Prevention in high-risk patients	Heparin 100 units/kg daily from day −9 to day +35
Supportive care in clinically significant VOD	Restrict fluids to 80% of maintenance
	Minimise sodium intake
	Maximise calorie intake
	Keep albumin >35 g/l with 20% albumin solution
	Use diuretics
	Maintain normal plasma potassium
	Ensure adequate analgesia (opiates are often required)
	Paracentesis for discomfort, respiratory difficulty and oliguria associated with ascites
	Early liaison with intensive care unit and consideration of continuous positive airways pressure
Specific therapy in severe disease	Anti-thrombin III to maintain level >120%: during first 24 hours 50 units/kg 8-hourly, then 50 units/kg 24-hourly; continue for 10 days
	Do not co-prescribe heparin Defibrotide

Drug therapy

A wide range of drugs have been used to prevent VOD. In particular, low-dose heparin 100 units/kg daily has been shown to be safe and to reduce the incidence of VOD in a single randomised trial, but heparin failed to prevent severe VOD in very high-risk patients in another study. Prostaglandin E1 reduces platelet aggregation and is a vasodilator that may reduce the incidence of VOD, but it has unacceptable toxicity. There is no evidence of any benefit from the use of oxpentifylline (pentoxyfylline). Very early results from Morris in Cincinnati suggest that continuous infusion

of anti-thrombin III may prevent occlusive disease, but there are no data from randomised prospective studies. Our current practice is to identify patients at high risk of VOD according to the criteria shown in Box 3.5 and to administer low-dose continuous heparin from 9 days before until 35 days after BMT.

Simple anticoagulation with full-dose heparin has no role in the treatment of progressive disease, and the results of the use of prostaglandin E_1 are mixed, but the utility of the latter is limited by toxicity. The administration of r-tPA has been investigated extensively by Bearman and colleagues in Seattle and Denver. Because of concerns over the risk of fatal haemorrhage associated with r-tPA, only patients deemed to have greater than 40% risk of death from VOD (as defined by a statistical model) were given the drug. A total of 42 patients were treated, 30 of whom already required dialysis or mechanical ventilation prior to therapy, and 12 responded. Severe bleeding was seen in ten patients; three of these died as direct consequence and bleeding was implicated in the death of a further three. The authors recommended that r-tPA should not be administered to patients with VOD who have developed multiorgan failure. Unfortunately, this is the very group who are candidates for more aggressive therapy. One logical conclusion of this study is to intervene earlier. However, we do not believe that there is sufficient evidence for the efficacy of this drug to risk potentially fatal bleeding in patients whose VOD may resolve with supportive management alone.

A more recently described intervention is the use of anti-thrombin III. Morris *et al.* have suggested that this is an effective and safe treatment of established VOD. In a non-randomised study 10 children with progressive clinically significant VOD and other organ dysfunction, who had anti-thrombin III levels below 88 IU/l, received anti-thrombin III concentrate to maintain a level of greater than 120% for 3–12 days. Clinical improvement was seen in all patients and the probability of death caused by VOD and organ dysfunction was significantly reduced when compared with historic controls. The value of anti-thrombin III has yet to be confirmed in a prospective randomised study.

Very recent data from Richardson *et al.* suggest a role for the polydeoxyribonucleotide Defibrotide in severe VOD. This agent is increasingly widely used and may be equivalent or better than ATIII. We have no direct experience of this drug and the reader is referred to the original article for dose schedules.

Our current policy for the treatment of progressive disease is shown in Table 3.4. This type of intervention is reserved for patients with respiratory embarrassment caused by ascites, those with rapid early weight gain and rise in bilirubin or those with evidence of pulmonary involvement. We currently eschew the use of thrombolytics. There are several reports of the successful use of liver transplantation in patients with VOD after BMT. However, as synthetic failure of the liver is a late event in this process and is normally preceded by pulmonary and renal failure, the utility of this approach is limited.

Post-transplant immunodeficiency

Immune reconstitution following a non T-cell-depleted matched sibling (MSD) BMT is relatively rapid and adequate T-cell numbers (CD4 count >0.3 × 10^9 cells/l) and function can be demonstrated at 6 months in most patients. By contrast, immune reconstitution after transplants from alternative donors is much slower. Severe T-cell lymphopenia has been described up to 2 years following T-cell-depleted unrelated BMT in adults. It must also be remembered that patients who receive high-dose therapy are considered to be functionally asplenic.

Each transplant unit should have clear strategies for the prevention of opportunistic infection, irradiation of blood products to prevent transfusion-associated GvHD and for eventual re-immunization. Education of patients, their parents and medical and nursing staff as to the risks associated with immunodeficiency is integral to the success of such an approach. Facilities must be available for rapid re-admission of post-transplant patients for investigation of fever (see below). Regular monitoring of immune reconstitution (lymphocyte subsets, serum immunoglobulins and phytohaemagglutinin response) should be undertaken. Only when adequate reconstitution is documented should the prophylactic regimen be withdrawn. It is hoped that this approach will minimise the incidence of late opportunistic infection. An obvious caveat is the absence of tests of specific immunity and there is no substitute for clinical vigilance.

Cytomegalovirus and pneumocystic infection

Widespread adoption of anti-viral prophylaxis, allied to sensitive methods for detection of reactivation of viruses and early intervention with ganciclovir, has radically reduced the impact of CMV on early transplant-related mortality. *Pneumocystis carinii* pneumonia (PCP) can be prevented by the use of low-dose cotrimoxazole and we have never seen PCP in patients who are reliably taking this drug. Prophylactic cotrimoxazole should be given from the date of admission until day 1 after BMT and recommenced on count recovery. An alternative is pentamidine (Table 3.5) but breakthrough infection can occur in patients receiving this drug and it must be considered inferior to cotrimoxazole.

Aspergillosis

Invasive aspergillosis is the most common cause of death in the first 100 days after BMT. Although there is as yet no proven method for the prevention of this infection, we attempt to reduce the risk of *Aspergillus* infection by early prophylaxis with oral itraconazole. The drug should be started at least 1 month prior to conditioning to ensure adequate tissue loading prior to the procedure. Itraconazole is associated with the development of transaminitis in a minority of patients and in these children fluconazole or amphotericin should be employed (Table 3.5). Establishing a firm diagnosis of fungal infection is difficult. Serological markers are not reliable. Potentially dangerous invasive procedures such as bronchoalveolar lavage or liver biopsy may fail to reveal the presence of *Aspergillus*, which is subsequently documented at postmortem. Therefore, in most patients, the institution of aggressive antifungal therapy must be empiric. Nephrotoxicity of conventional amphotericin is often aggravated in children receiving cyclosporin, and as there is now good evidence that lipid formulations of amphotericin are at least equally effective and better tolerated, these should be used as first-line treatment in BMT patients.

Respiratory viral infections

Respiratory viruses (particularly myxoviruses) are emerging as major pathogens in the post-transplant

Table 3.5 Protocol for prevention of infection after BMT	
Infection	**Treatment**
Cytomegalovirus: prevention	Blood and platelets should be obtained from CMV negative donors (leucodepletion to a guaranteed leucocyte count of 1×10^6 cells/l is an acceptable alternative)
Low-risk patients (recipient and donor CMV negative)	Intravenous acyclovir 250 mg/m^2 three times a day. From day −5 change to 300 mg/m^2 four times a day and to oral doses at day +28; in the absence of chronic GvHD continue for 6 months
High-risk patients (either recipient or donor or both CMV positive)	Intravenous acyclovir 500 mg/m^2 three times a day. From day −5 convert to 600 mg/m^2 four times a day and to oral doses at day +28; in the absence of chronic GvHD continue for 6 months
Very-high-risk patients (previous infection or excreting CMV prior to BMT)	Intravenous ganciclovir 5 mg/kg twice daily from day −10 to day −1; restart at neutrophils >0.5 × 10^9 cells/l. Switch to acyclovir when CMV PCR negative for 14 days; in the absence of chronic GvHD continue acyclovir for 6 months
Cytomegalovirus: reactivation	
Early detection of reactivation	Twice weekly buffy coat for antigenaemia (or clinically validated PCR)
Treatment of reactivation	Ganciclovir 5mg/kg until antigenaemia resolves; then 5mg/kg daily for 1 week
Fungi: prevention	Oral itraconazole syrup 5 mg/kg. Start fluconazole (3 mg/kg) if itraconazole stopped. Stop itraconazole/fluconazole when ANC >1 × 10^9 cells/l except if acute GvHD or on steroids
Humoral immunodeficiency: treatment	Weekly intravenous gammaglobulin (0.5 g/kg) started on admission. In immunodeficiency or in the presence of acute GvHD continue 3-weekly until recovery of IgM and IgA. In matched related grafts stop on discharge. In matched unrelated and haploidentical transplants continue till CD4 >300 × 10^6 cells/l
Pneumocystis carinii: prevention	Septrin until day −1 regardless of neutrophil count. Restart septrin post-transplant when ANC is >0.5 × 10^9 cells/l. Continue for a minimum of 6 months or until cyclosporin is stopped or PHA response normal. Use pentamidine nebuliser 4-weekly or intravenous 2-weekly in patients unable to tolerate septrin
Capsular bacterial sepsis: prevention	Penicillin or alternative prophylaxis from day 28 (assess for penicillin resistance); vaccination against *Haemophilus influenza* B
Other viruses	Revaccinate as per recommendations (Box 3.3)

ANC, absolute neutrophil count; PCR, polymerase chain reaction.

period. Two distinct, but not exclusive, patterns of infection are seen. Respiratory syncytial virus (RSV) leads to a devastating primary viral pneumonia. By contrast influenza and parainfluenza are more commonly limited to the upper respiratory tract or associated with a self-limiting pneumonic illness; severe pneumonia is often associated with secondary bacterial infection in these patients.

The morbidity and mortality of RSV infection can be significantly reduced if spread to the lower respiratory tract is prevented (Fig. 3.2). As infection is often secondary to asymptomatic carriage prior to BMT, a nasopharyngeal aspirate should be obtained in all patients on the day of admission. If RSV is detected then it would be prudent to defer the procedure. When this is not possible, or if RSV is isolated from the upper respiratory tract during the transplant course, then ribavirin and hyperimmune globulin (Respigam) should be administered. There is no evidence that ribavirin significantly delays engraftment.

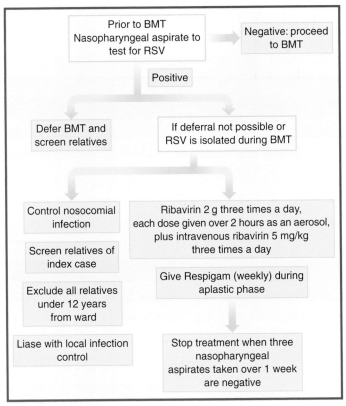

Figure 3.2 *Management of RSV infection in BMT patients. Nosocomial infection is minimised by screening relatives of index case.*

Unfortunately pneumonia may be the first manifestation of RSV infection in up to 25% of patients, and even with anti-viral therapy the mortality is greater than 80% in most series. RSV is highly contagious and may spread rapidly throughout a transplant unit. Aggressive policies for the prevention of nosocomial infection have been shown to reduce the incidence of RSV disease during outbreaks in major units. Our policy for RSV is currently extended to patients colonised with other respiratory viruses.

Adenoviruses cause upper respiratory tract and gastrointestinal infection in children and reactivation of latent virus or primary infection has now been widely described after BMT. Serotypes belonging to subgroups B and C are most commonly isolated. Several patterns of adenoviral infection are recognised. Incidental detection in an asymptomatic patient is increasingly common with the institution of specific screening. Primary gastrointestinal infection may lead to severe diarrhoea and must be differentiated from GvHD. Biopsy may be of value in this context. Adenovirus has also been implicated in the development of haemorrhagic cystitis. Of greater

concern is the increasing number of reports of disseminated adenoviral infection. Some of these children appear simply to develop a rapidly fatal fulminant hepatitis (liver failure can supervene within 72 hours of the first abnormal liver function tests), often accompanied by pneumonitis. In others there is a prodromal diarrhoeal illness that may be treated as GvHD. Then, days to weeks later, there is evidence of rapidly progressive liver dysfunction or pneumonitis. To date, there are no evidence-based guidelines for the management of adenoviral infection after BMT. Whereas vidaribine and ganciclovir appear to be effective in haemorrhagic cystitis, specific anti-viral therapy of other sites of established infection is unsatisfactory. Isolated gastrointestinal disease may respond to oral immunoglobulin and supportive management. Disseminated adenovirus is normally fatal, and although treatment with ribavirin is widely employed there is no evidence that it is of benefit.

As with other infections in the transplant recipient prevention is preferable to treatment. Surveillance microbiological screening should be used to alert the physician to the possibility of adenoviral infection. It is possible that dissemination of adenovirus may be encouraged by further immunosuppression, and so biopsy confirmation of GvHD should be sought in patients with suggestive symptoms prior to therapy in the presence of intercurrent adenovirus infection. Liver biopsy may be associated with uncontrolled haemorrhage in fulminant adenoviral hepatitis and is contraindicated.

The emergence of adenoviruses and respiratory viruses as significant pathogens in recipients of allogeneic transplants may simply reflect improvements in prophylaxis against CMV and *P. carinii*. However, these infections are more common in recipients of alternative donor transplants. It is this group of patients who have prolonged immunodeficiency and may require continued immunosuppression. This is particularly relevant as we move toward an era in which the absence of a suitably matched donor can be overcome by the use of profoundly T-cell-depleted haploidentical grafts. At present, it seems that immunodeficiency rather than GvHD or graft failure may be the limiting toxicity of these procedures. The early 21st century will see the development of anti-viral T-cell clones and specifically engineered grafts. Adoptive immunotherapy has already been successfully used to treat adenoviral infection after BMT.

Further reading

Bearman, S.I. (1995) The syndrome of hepatic veno-occlusive disease after marrow transplantation. *Blood* 85: 3005–3020.

Hann, I., Viscoli, C., Paesmans, M., Gaya, H. and Glauser, M. (1997) A comparison of outcome from febrile neutropenic episodes in children compared with adults: results from four EORTC studies. *British Journal of Haematology* 99: 580–588.

Mitchell, L.G., Sutor, A.H. and Andrew, M. (1995) Haemostasis in childhood acute lymphoblastic leukaemia: coagulopathy induced by disease and treatment. *Seminars in Thrombosis and Haemostasis* 21: 390–401.

Morris, J.D., Harris, R.E., Hashmi, R. *et al.* (1997) Antithrombin-III for the treatment of chemotherapy-induced organ dysfunction following bone marrow transplantation. *Bone Marrow Transplantation* 20: 871–878.

Prentice, H.G., Kho, P. (1997) Clinical strategies for the management of cytomegalovirus infection and disease in allogeneic bone marrow transplant. *Bone Marrow Transplantation* 19: 135–142.

Richardson, P., Elias, A., Krishnan, A. *et al.* (1998) Treatment of severe veno-occlusive disease with Defibrotide: compassionate use results in response without significant toxicity in a high risk population. *Blood* 92: 737–744.

Sparrelid, E., Ljungman, P., Ekelof-Andstrom, E. *et al.* (1997) Ribavirin therapy in bone marrow transplant recipients with viral respiratory tract infections. *Bone Marrow Transplantation* 19: 905–908.

Wheeler, K., Chessells, J.H., Bailey, C.C. and Richards, S.M. (1996) Treatment related deaths during induction and first remission in acute lymphoblastic leukaemia. *Archives of Disease in Childhood* 74: 101–107.

CHAPTER 4

Non-Hodgkin's lymphoma

C.R. Pinkerton

Introduction

The outcome for patients with non-Hodgkin's lymphoma (NHL) has improved dramatically with intensive chemotherapy. Interest has, therefore, focussed on some of the less common subtypes, such as anaplastic large cell, peripheral T-cell and immunodeficiency-related lymphoproliferative disorders. A continuing problem in paediatric NHL is terminology. As with adult NHL, there is a history of multiple histopathological groupings, which have led to considerable confusion when it comes to comparing clinical data. The recent French–American–British collaboration in childhood NHL has taken the decision to apply the REAL (Revised European American Lymphoma) classification in order to try to standardise terminology between three national groups. The relevant subgroups of the REAL classification are outlined in Table 4.1.

The REAL classification is an extension of the Kiel classification, arranging tumours on the basis of immunophenotype. The extensive array of monoclonal antibodies identifying the B and T lineage of lymphoblasts usually facilitates allocation. In some situations, this may be difficult and molecular analysis documenting patterns of immunoglobulin gene or T-cell receptor gene rearrangements are of value. In the more difficult cases where both markers and molecular studies are ambiguous, the most reliable contribution is from an experienced histopathologist, taking into account the pattern of clinical presentation (Fig. 4.1).

Documentation of cytogenetic alterations and patterns of gene rearrangement may also prove to be of

Table 4.1 The REAL classification			
Cell type		Subgroups	Proportion of NHL (%)
B cell	I	Precursor B neoplasm	
		B lymphoblastic	5
	II	Peripheral B neoplasm	
		Follicular	0.4
		Diffuse large B cell	3
		Primary mediastinal (sclerosing)	0.4
		Burkitt's	42
		High-grade B; Burkitt-like	4
T cell	I	Precursor T neoplasm T lymphoblastic	20
	II	Peripheral T cell	
		PTL unspecified	1
		Anaplastic large cell	15
		Non-specific/indeterminate	9.2

value in the detection of minimal residual disease at the time of apparent complete clinical remission. The evaluation of this runs in parallel with larger studies in ALL.

The largest subgroups are the peripheral B neoplasms: Burkitt and Burkitt-like. Dramatic improvements in cure rate for these tumours have come with increased doses and dose intensity of conventional drugs such as cyclophosphamide, methotrexate and cytarabine. While somewhat poorer, the outcome of precursor T lymphoblastic lymphomas is comparable to that for ALL at around 70% event-free survival at 5 years.

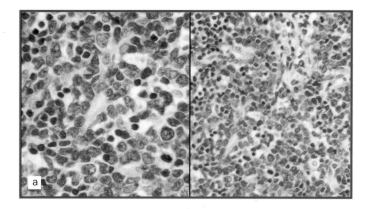

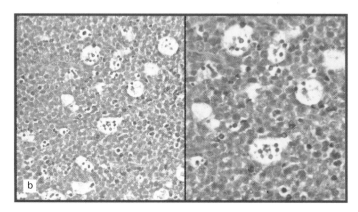

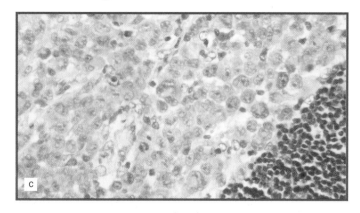

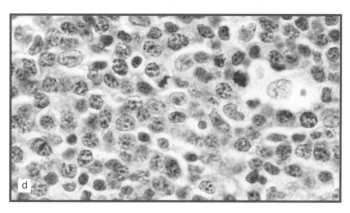

Figure 4.1 *Histological features of subgroups of NHL. (a) Lymphoblastic T-cell; (b) Burkitt's; (c) anaplastic large cell; (d) lymphoblastoid 'lymphoma' subsequent to liver transplant.*

Staging

The Murphy staging system is generally accepted for paediatric NHL and has, in the past, served well to predict outcome and stratify patients for treatment (Table 4.2). Chest X-ray and ultrasound examination are sufficient to document the presence of disease in the chest and abdomen in the majority of patients. Increasingly, CT scan or MRI is used as a routine for initial staging, but these should probably be reserved for those patients in whom chest X-ray and ultrasound are negative. Precise delineation of nodal involvement above or below the diaphragm is not critical, as Stages II–IV all receive intensive chemotherapy (Figs. 4.2–4.4). Only in Stage I patients is CT required to exclude nodal involvement outside the main site of disease. Similarly,

Table 4.2 The Murphy staging system	
Stage	Characteristics
I	A single tumour (extranodal) or single anatomical area (nodal), with the exclusion of the mediastinum or abdomen
II	A single tumour (extranodal) with regional node involvement
	Two or more nodal areas on the same side of the diaphragm
	Two single (extranodal) tumours with or without regional node involvement on the same side of the diaphragm
	A primary gastrointestinal tract tumour, usually in the ileocaecal area, with or without involvement of associated mesenteric nodes only, grossly completely resected
III	Two single tumours (extranodal) on opposite sides of the diaphragm
	Two or more nodal areas above and below the diaphragm
	All the primary intrathoracic tumours (mediastinal, pleural, thymic)
	All extensive primary intra-abdominal disease, unresectable
	All paraspinal or epidural tumours, regardless of other tumour site(s)
IV	Any of the above with initial CNS and/or bone marrow involvement

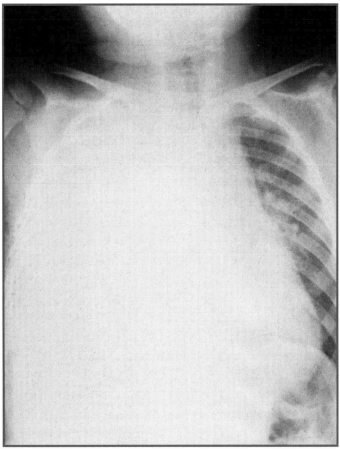

Figure 4.2 *Large mediastinal T-cell lymphoma, causing white-out of hemithorax.*

although high-dose gallium or, more recently, PET (positron emission tomography) scanning may be used to detect the precise extent of disease, these contribute little to the overall management of the patient. Recent analyses of outcome have indicated that (lactic dehydrogenase) LDH is one of the more important prognostic factors and this has been incorporated into risk group stratification. Another factor is the extent of bone marrow involvement. The French SFOP group consider the risk of CNS disease to be significantly higher if there are more than 70% blast cells in the marrow or there are circulating blast cells; these patients are treated with a more intensive B-ALL regimen.

For anaplastic large cell lymphoma, the Murphy staging system is probably inappropriate. The majority fall into Murphy stage III, which does not give any real indication of the likely outcome. As discussed below, it is becoming increasingly apparent that other clinical factors will indicate outcome, and a novel staging system is required.

Issues regarding management of specific types of NHL

Precursor T-cell lymphoblastic lymphoma
There is now a consensus that precursor T-cell lymphoblastic lymphoma behaves in a similar

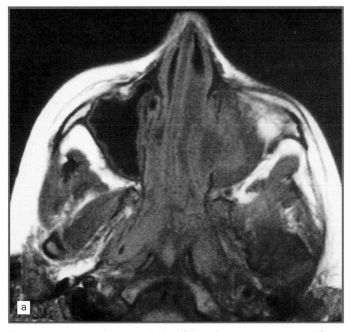
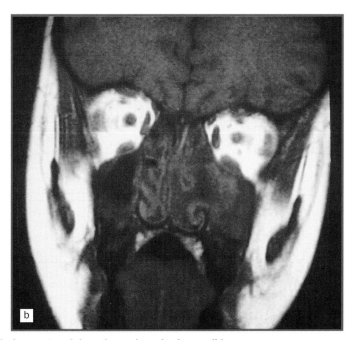

Figure 4.3 *Nasopharyngeal B-cell lymphoma presenting with nasal obstruction (a) and purulent discharge (b).*

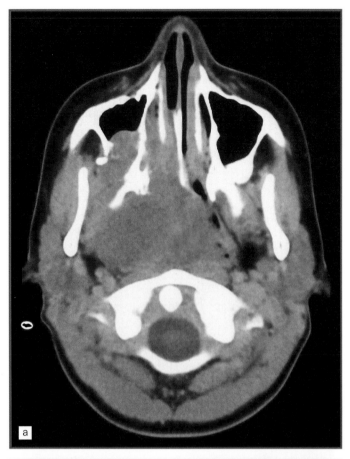

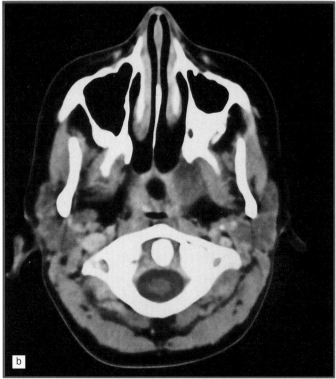

Figure 4.4 *Large nasopharyngeal B-cell lymphoma (a) at initial presentation with pharyngeal obstruction; (b) repeat scan within 4 weeks of commencing intensive chemotherapy.*

fashion to T-cell lymphoblastic leukaemia and is biologically close, if not identical. Non-localised disease is treated with prolonged chemotherapy, involving induction, consolidation and up to 2 years continuing chemotherapy. The treatment of localised tumours is more contentious. The current UKCCSG strategy is to treat these with an identical protocol to that used for non-localised disease. The POG randomised study of COMP versus the LSA2 L2 protocol contained too few localised tumours to indicate whether the short regimen was adequate. Anecdotal experience in the UK using a CHOP-based regimen for Stage I and II precursor T-cell lymphoblastic lymphomas revealed a high incidence of marrow and CNS relapse. The inconvenience of prolonged leukaemia-type treatment and the potential morbidity related to anthracyclines or etoposide must be taken into consideration but, conversely, the omission of cyclophosphamide is an advantage with regard to male fertility.

It has proved difficult to delineate clinical prognostic features in this tumour type and initial bulk of disease does not appear to be of significance. Slow responders have a higher failure rate and in the current UKCCSG regimen, additional early intensification of chemotherapy is given to patients who fail to achieve radiological complete remission after the first 6 weeks of chemotherapy. The role of radiotherapy remains debatable. A single randomised study indicated superior outcome for those who received involved field radiotherapy but with current more intensive leukaemia-based chemotherapy this is probably not necessary. It may, however, have a role to play in some refractory cases with only localised disease.

CNS-directed therapy

In the past, cranial irradiation was used. It seems likely that, as in ALL, either intrathecal methotrexate alone or combined with pulses of high-dose methotrexate are comparable. There are no randomised studies to confirm this in NHL, but analysis of sequential series in the UK has indicated that a change from cranial irradiation to high-dose methotrexate was not associated with any significant increase in CNS relapse rate.

Precursor B-cell lymphoblastic lymphoma

The B lymphoblastic lymphomas may be either CD10 positive or cytoplasmic μ positive, equivalent to solid deposits of common ALL or pre-B ALL. Treatment is as for precursor B lineage leukaemia, irrespective of the extent of initial disease. As with precursor T disease, there seems little doubt that if these children are treated with reduced chemotherapy (e.g. CHOP-based regimens) the relapse rate will be higher.

Peripheral B-cell lymphoma (Burkitt and Burkitt-like)

How intensive treatment regimens need to be for the peripheral B lymphomas remains a subject of debate. Dramatic improvement in outcome has been associated with a significant escalation of dose and dose intensity. It seems possible that some subgroups are currently being overtreated and the children subjected to unnecessarily high risks of sterilisation, cardiac toxicity and second malignancy. It is, however, difficult to reduce highly effective treatment, which is moderately well tolerated in terms of acute morbidity. At the present time in the UK, children on the FAB LMB regimen with Stage I disease are given very short treatment, namely, two courses of COPAd. Stages II–IV disease receive the more intensive COPAdM-CyM regimen and those with CNS disease or B-ALL have consolidation with a high dose cytosine arabinoside (AraC)/etoposide regimen. There is some continued debate regarding Stage I and II patients, as to whether the late sequelae of anthracyclines are more important to avoid than the sterilising effect of cyclophosphamide. In the recent UKCCSG study, cyclosphosphamide was omitted from a CHOP-based regimen, with no apparent adverse effect on outcome.

The rarer large B-cell lymphoma should be treated as for Burkitt's lymphoma, and outcome is comparable. The one difference is that with the sclerosing mediastinal B-cell tumours, local irradiation should be considered if there is a slow response to chemotherapy.

Which patients need CNS irradiation?

In the past, all children presenting with either blast cells in the CSF or evidence of leptomeningeal disease received craniospinal irradiation and, more recently, cranial irradiation alone. The dramatic improvement in outcome for these children followed the introduction of more intensive triple intrathecal therapy and high-dose cytosine, the previous outcome having been very poor despite aggressive irradiation. It seems likely that CNS irradiation is not necessary and in the current FAB LMB study, control of CNS disease relies on high-dose cytarabine, high-dose methotrexate and repeated intrathecal triple therapy. There is still justification for craniospinal irradiation in relapsed patients, where it can be included as a boost with total body irradiation or precede high-dose chemotherapy with stem cell rescue.

Speed of response

Peripheral B lymphoma is an exquisitely chemosensitive tumour and often patients are in complete remission within 3–4 weeks of starting chemotherapy. Response to an initial pre-phase with COP has not proved to be a significant prognostic factor but patients who fail to achieve a complete remission by the end of 10–12 weeks of chemotherapy have, in the past, had a higher recurrence rate. A strategy for these patients is outlined in Figure 4.5.

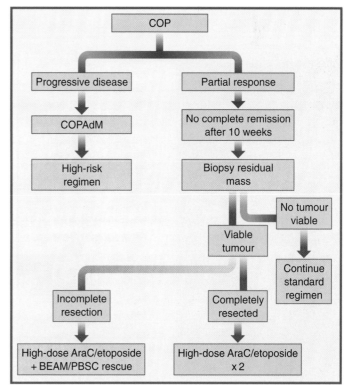

Figure 4.5 *Algorithm for management of poor responders with B-NHL.*

Anaplastic large cell lymphoma

Anaplastic large cell lymphoma (ALCL) now makes up almost one fifth of childhood NHL. The increased awareness of this group has come with more sophisticated immunophenotyping. Characteristic features include CD30 and EMA positivity and in many cases a t(2;5) translocation (Fig. 4.6). The precise incidence of this translocation is at present unclear, estimates varying depending on the method used. The use of FISH (fluorescence *in situ* hybridisation), and more recently the detection of the aberrant transcript using either monoclonal antibody (ALK) or RT-PCR (reverse transcriptase–polymerase chain reaction), has increased the detection rate. Some published data continue to include CD30-negative tumours as part of ALCL, but the UK policy has been to restrict this tumour type to CD30-positive samples. With adequate immunohistochemistry CD30-negative tumours that are morphologically ALCL are extremely rare. Whether the t(2;5) translocation tumours reflect a subgroup that behaves differently remains to be demonstrated, although anecdotal reports have suggested that the Hodgkin's-like variant may be ALK negative. The lymphohistiocytic type is said to have a poor prognosis, but the incidence of this subgroup remains to be clearly defined.

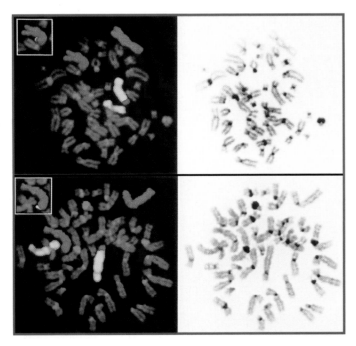

Figure 4.6 *t(2;5) translocation in anaplastic large cell lymphoma. Chromosome 2 = red; chromosome 5 = yellow.*

What staging system should be used?

As mentioned above, the Murphy system is inappropriate for ALCL, as almost all will be Stage III (Fig. 4.7). A recent collaborative analysis of ALCL patients in Europe has revealed three prognostic subgroups. Patients with mediastinal disease and skin involvement do particularly poorly, with only around 10–20% disease-free survival (DFS). An intermediate group, with approximately 50% DFS have either skin or mediastinum involvement, in addition to other nodal or extranodal sites, and a third low-risk group (DFS approximately 80%), with no skin, mediastinal or lung parenchymal involvement. It is hoped that a new collaborative European study, using a standard chemotherapy protocol, will enable the development of a novel prognostically useful staging system.

Slow response in ALCL appears to be less important than in high-grade B lymphomas, and these tumours may behave more like Hodgkin's disease. Assessment of complete remission can wait until the end of chemotherapy but if there is residual imageable mass at that time this should be biopsied. As in Hodgkin's disease, residual nodal disease at this stage may benefit from local radiotherapy. High unremitting fevers are a characteristic symptom in ALCL, which usually respond to initial steroid-containing chemotherapy. In some cases, this symptom may be very severe, particularly at the time of disease relapse.

What is the role of high-dose chemotherapy and stem cell rescue in childhood lymphoma?

Several years ago many patients with advanced disease, either B- or T-NHL, were electively allografted or autografted in complete remission. This is now clearly inappropriate and in pre-T lymphomas, allografting should be restricted to patients with early relapses less than 2 years from presentation, particularly where there is marrow involvement. A late nodal or mediastinal recurrence may benefit from high-dose therapy and autograft, possibly with mediastinal radiotherapy, although this is not of proved value.

With Burkitt's peripheral B-cell lymphoma, allografting is indicated where there is an early bone marrow relapse or disease progression at any site on therapy. For local relapses, autografting may again be

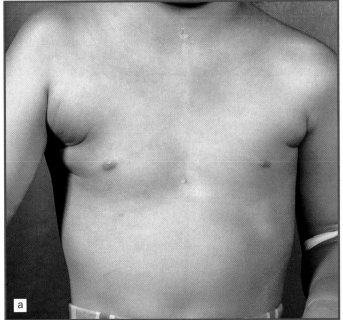

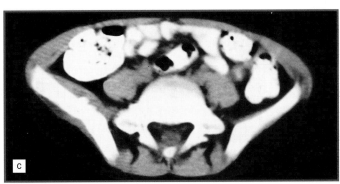

appropriate. Figures 4.8 and 4.9 give algorithms for treatment of relapsed pre-T or pre-B NHL and for Burkitt's or Burkitt-like lymphoma, respectively.

Management of relapsed ALCL poses a major problem. Although both autografting and allografting have been used in the past, there is little real evidence to support their efficacy. Second-line regimens appropriate for high-grade lymphoma, for example protocols incorporating high-dose AraC, are probably not particularly effective, but impressive responses have been achieved using Hodgkin's regimens, for example ChlVPP or even single-agent weekly vinblastine (Fig. 4.10).

There is particular interest in the increasing problem of immunosuppression/immunodeficiency-related lymphoproliferative disorders, particularly after organ or marrow transplant and HIV. Registers to

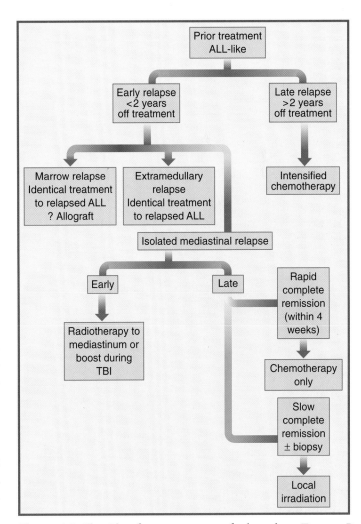

Figure 4.7 *Anaplastic large cell lymphoma. (a) Typical subcutaneous infiltration; (b) parenchymal lung involvement; (c) soft tissue mass adjacent to bony lesion.*

Figure 4.8 *Algorithm for management of relapsed pre-T or pre-B NHL.*

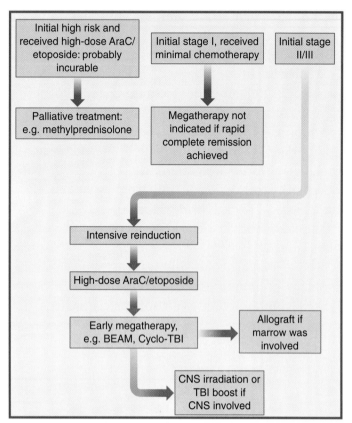

Figure 4.9 *Algorithm for management of relapsed Burkitt/Burkitt-like lymphoma.*

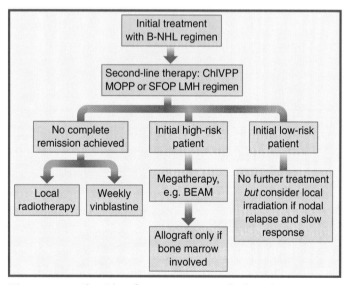

Figure 4.10 *Algorithm for management of relapsed ALCL.*

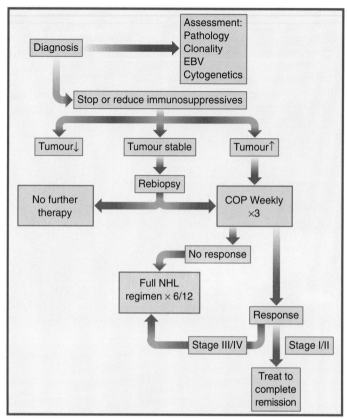

Figure 4.11 *Algorithm for management of post-transplant lymphoproliferative disease. COP, cyclophosphamide, vincristine and prednisolone.*

document the nature of this problem have been set up in the UK and USA. A scheme for management of post-transplant lymphoproliferative disease (PTLD) is shown in Figure 4.11. Withdrawal or reduction of immunosuppression is a delicate matter and will depend on the transplant type. Earlier use of chemotherapy could reduce mortality in some patients but clinical and biological parameters to guide this decision remain unclear. Novel strategies such as use of interleukin-2 and adoptive immunotherapy with EBV-specific T-cells are currently under evaluation.

Further reading

Avet-Loiseau, H., Hartmann, O., Valteau, D. *et al.* (1991) High-dose chemotherapy containing busulfan followed by bone marrow transplantation in 24 children with refractory or relapsed non-Hodgkin's lymphoma. *Bone Marrow Transplant* 8: 465–472.

Bowman, W.P., Shuster, J., Cook, B. *et al.* (1996) Improved survival for children with B cell (SIg⁺) acute lymphoblastic leukemia and stage IV small non-cleaved cell lymphoma: a POG study. *Journal of Clinical Oncology* 14: 1252–1261.

Eden, O., Hann, I., Imeson, J. *et al.* (1992) Treatment of advanced stage T cell lymphoblastic lymphoma: results of the United Kingdom Children's Cancer Study Group (UKCCSG) protocol 8503. *British Journal of Haematology* 82: 310–316.

Gentet, J.C., Patte, C., Quintana, E. *et al.* (1990) Phase II study of cytarabine and etoposide in children with refractory or relapsed non-Hodgkin's lymphoma: a study of the French Society of Pediatric Oncology, *Journal of Clinical Oncology* 8: 661–665.

Gerritsen, E.J.A., Stam, E.D., Hermans, J. *et al.* (1990) Risk factors for developing EBV-related B cell lymphoproliferative disorders (BLPD) after non-HLA-identical BMT in children. *Bone Marrow Transplant* 18: 377–382.

Hutchison, R.E., Berard, C.W., Shuster, J.J. *et al.* (1995) B-cell lineage confers a favorable outcome among children and adolescents with large cell lymphoma: a Pediatric Oncology Group study. *Journal of Clinical Oncology* 13: 2023–2032.

Niedobitek,G. and Young, L.S. (1994) Epstein–Barr virus persistence and virus-associated tumours. *Lancet* 343: 333–335.

Patte, C., Philip, T., Rodary, C. *et al.* (1991) High survival rate in advanced stage B-cell lymphomas and leukemias without CNS involvement with a short intensive polychemotherapy. Results of a randomized trial from the French Pediatric Oncology Society (SFOP) on 216 children. *Journal of Clinical Oncology* 9: 123–132.

Philip, T., Hartmann, O., Michon, J. *et al.* (1993) Curability of relapsed childhood B-cell non-Hodgkin's lymphoma following intensive first line therapy. *Blood* 81: 2003–2006.

Pinkerton, C.R., Hann, I., Eden, O.B. *et al.* (1991) Outcome in stage III non-Hodgkin's lymphoma in children (UKCCSG study NHL 86). How much treatment is needed? *British Journal of Cancer* 64: 583–587.

Reiter, A., Schrappe, M., Parwaresch, R. *et al.* (1995) Non-Hodgkin's lymphomas of childhood and adolescence: results of a treatment stratified for biologic subtypes and stage. A report of the Berlin–Frankfurt–Munster Group. *Journal of Clinical Oncology* 13: 359–372.

Sandlund, J.T., Downing, J.R. and Crist, W.M. (1996) Non-Hodgkin's lymphoma in childhood. *New England Journal of Medicine* 334: 1238–1248.

Sandlund, J.T., Pui, C.-H., Santana, V.M. *et al.* (1994) Clinical features and treatment outcome for children with CD30+ large cell non-Hodgkin's lymphoma. *Journal of Clinical Oncology* 12: 895–898.

Swerdlow, S.H. (1997) Post-transplant lymphoproliferative disorders: a working classification. *Current Diagnostic Pathology* 4: 28–35.

Tubergen, D.G., Krailo, M.D., Meadows, A.T. *et al.* (1995) Comparison of treatment regimens for pediatric lymphoblastic non-Hodgkin's lymphoma: a Children's Cancer Group study. *Journal of Clinical Oncology* 13: 1368–1376.

CHAPTER 5

Hodgkin's disease

C.R. Pinkerton

Introduction

Although Hodgkin's lymphoma is one of the most curable of children's cancers, the optimal combination therapy leading to maximal survival with minimal late morbidity remains controversial and the relative emphasis on chemotherapy versus radiotherapy differs between national groups.

As with a number of other childhood cancers, the decision on therapy will depend on the investigator's perceived importance of differing toxicities and belief in the likelihood of cure with second-line chemotherapy. Initial treatment options are summarised in Table 5.1 and range from local irradiation to the involved field for Stage IA patients, as currently used in the UKCCSG, to intensive multiagent combination regimens combined with irradiation to multiple sites of disease, as in the German regimen for Stage IV disease.

The traditional Ann Arbor staging system continues to be used in paediatric practice (Table 5.2) but with

Table 5.1 Initial treatment options for Hodgkin's disease

Stage	Options
I/IIA	Local irradiation only or standard chemotherapy[a] alone or chemotherapy + irradiation
IIIA	Standard chemotherapy or hybrid[b] ± irradiation
IIIB or IV	Hybrid chemotherapy or COPP–OPPA + local irradiation ± multisite irradiation

[a] Chemotherapy: MOPP, ChlVPP, ABVD, VEEP.

[b] Hybrid treatment: ABVD + MOPP, ABVD + ChlVPP.

Table 5.2 Ann Arbor staging classification

Stage	Characteristics
I	Involvement of a single lymph node region (I) or a single extralymphatic organ or site (IE)
II	Involvement of two or more lymph node regions on the same side of the diaphragm (II) or solitary involvement of an extralymphatic organ or site and of one or more lymph node region on the same side of the diaphragm (IIE)
III	Involvement of lymph node regions on both sides of the diaphragm (III), which may be accompanied by localised involvement of extralymphatic organ or site (IIIE) or by involvement of the spleen (IIIS) or both (IIISE)
IV	Diffuse or disseminated involvement of one or more extralymphatic organs or tissues with or without associated lymph node enlargement

hybrid chemotherapy and involved-field radiotherapy there is little difference in outcome for Stages I–III, with only Stage IV continuing to have a significantly poorer outcome. There is a need to try to identify subgroups within these stages where the prognosis is either particularly good and treatment intensity can be reduced, or less good where the current combined modality approaches are justified and need to be improved.

Does pathology influence outcome?

Studies in adults have suggested that pathology significantly influences outcome but these data are complicated by differing treatment approaches. There is little doubt that the lymphocyte predominant subgroup does well and the lymphocyte depleted does poorly, but these subgroups make up only a small proportion of patients (Fig. 5.1). In childhood Hodgkin's disease, the relative percentage of the different subgroups varies widely among national studies, for reasons that are unclear but may reflect the differences in pathological definitions. A recent analysis of UKCCSG data has shown no significant difference between mixed cellularity (MC) and nodular sclerosing (NS) subtypes, except in the case of Stage IA treated with local radiotherapy, where there was a significantly worse outcome for those with mixed cellularity. It appears that this pathological subgroup is a more aggressive variant, in whom conservative local radiotherapy alone is not adequate (Fig. 5.2). Studies in adults indicating a difference in prognosis for type 1 versus type 2 nodular sclerosing (a definition reflecting the degree of lymphocyte infiltration) has not been confirmed in subsequent studies and, because of the excellent outcome in all patients with nodular sclerosing disease in childhood, it seems unlikely that a significant difference exists. In lymphocyte predominant (LP) nodular sclerosing Hodgkin's disease, where only a single node is involved, there is the possibility of surgery alone. This may be curative in this biologically indolent form and such an approach may be justified.

Management of the young child with Hodgkin's disease

There is little doubt that the treatment which is associated with highest failure-free survival is a combination of moderate-dose chemotherapy, such as MOPP or ABVD, with low-dose involved-field

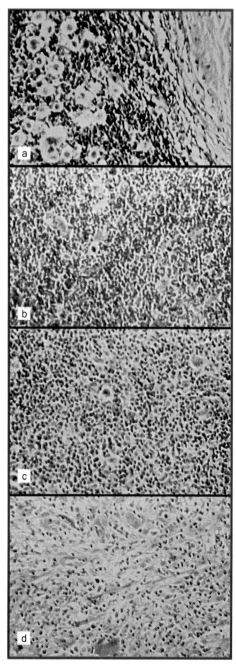

Figure 5.1 *Histological subtypes of Hodgkin's disease. (a) Mixed cellularity (MC, 32%); (b) nodular sclerosis (NS, 39%); (c) lymphocyte predominant (LP, 25%); (d) lymphocyte depleted (LD, 1%).*

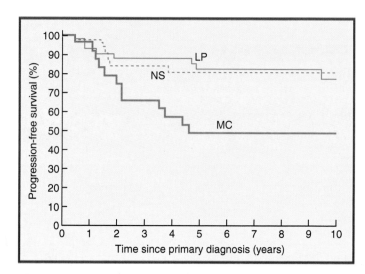

Figure 5.2 *Event-free survival for localised disease treated with irradiation alone in relation to histological subtype. NS, nodular sclerosing; MC, mixed cellularity; LP, lymphocyte predominant.*

irradiation. In the small child (i.e. less than 7 years) there may be concern about the use of local radiotherapy. Even doses as low as 20 Gy will probably be associated with soft tissue and bony undergrowth (Fig. 5.3). To what extent this is less than when 30–40 Gy are used remains contentious. It is in this group of young children where a chemotherapy alone strategy may be appropriate. For many years, the UKCCSG group has addressed the issue of chemotherapy alone as its main treatment strategy, except for high cervical Stage IA, where local irradiation is given. Six to eight courses of ChlVPP are associated with a relapse-free survival in excess of 80% for Stage II and IIIA patients, with an overall survival of over 90% for these groups. Up until recently, mediastinal irradiation was added for those with bulky mediastinal disease at presentation, i.e. greater than one-third the transthoracic diameter (Fig. 5.4). In the current national study, this has been dropped and the outcome of this non-randomised study is awaited to determine if this has adversely influenced relapse-free survival (Fig. 5.4). With this reservation about bulky mediastinal disease, it seems likely that an alkylating agent-based regimen alone will be sufficient to cure most children. The major reservation with this approach is that six to eight courses of such chemotherapy will invariably sterilise boys, almost certainly have an adverse effect on ovarian function in girls and may be associated in the long term with secondary malignancies, such as AML. For this reason,

a hybrid regimen may be attractive; however, this introduces the necessity to insert a central venous line for the administration of prolonged-infusion anthracycline and additional potential toxicities from the anthracycline and bleomycin. The VEEP regimen, which may have fewer late effects, has been evaluated in a limited number of patients, but the relapse rate is higher. There are few data regarding the activity of ABVD alone, but similar reservations have been expressed. Although the ultimate salvage rate in children who relapse having received VEEP is high, there is a worrying percentage who progress on initial treatment, in whom the salvage rate is poor. Data with other non-alkylating regimens such as ABVD without irradiation are limited. At present, the appropriate treatment for a smaller child with Stage II/III disease is probably a hybrid regimen, accepting that up to eight courses will have to be used if radiotherapy is to be avoided.

What approach should be taken for those with Stage IV or B symptoms? Analysis of UKCCSG data has shown that fewer than half the patients receiving ChlVPP with or without X-ray radiotherapy remain relapse-free at 5 years. Although a percentage of those relapsing will be salvaged with intensive second-line chemotherapy (Fig. 5.5), these results are inferior to those achieved by the German group and subsequently the SIOP group, using an identical regimen, shown in Table 5.3. This combines most of the active agents with extensive irradiation and is associated with a very high relapse-free survival. Careful analysis of the outcome with less intensive protocols, such as the UKCCSG approach, will reveal prognostic indicators and allow selection of which patients really require such intensive multimodality treatment.

Management of refractory or recurrent disease

Primary refractory Hodgkin's disease is extremely rare, even with initial advanced disease. The unusual primary refractory Stage I–III patient can change to second-line chemotherapy, which even if accompanied by a clear response should none the less be given with at least involved-field, if not extended-field, radiotherapy to consolidate initial remission. If there is

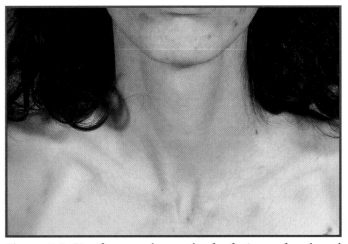

Figure 5.3 *Significant undergrowth of soft tissue of neck and clavicular region, secondary to mantle radiotherapy at a dose of 30 Gy.*

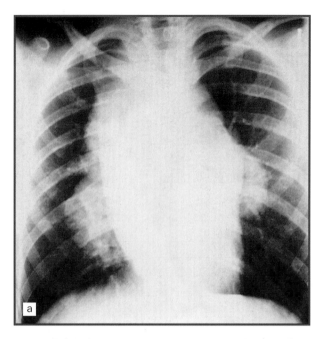

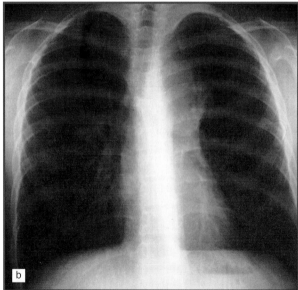

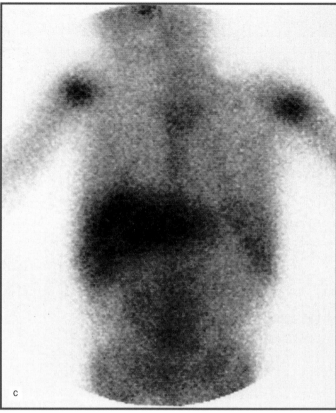

Figure 5.4 *Mediastinal mass. (a) Pre-therapy and (b) post-therapy. At the end of treatment significant residual widening of the upper mediastinum is apparent, which was positive on Gallium scan (c), indicating residual active disease.*

a slow response to second-line chemotherapy, then one should consider dose escalation and consolidation with megatherapy.

Patients with a late relapse, particularly those with initial localised disease, will usually respond to second-line chemotherapy plus involved-field radiotherapy, with a high salvage rate.

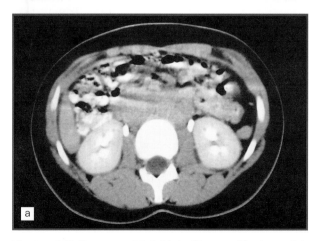

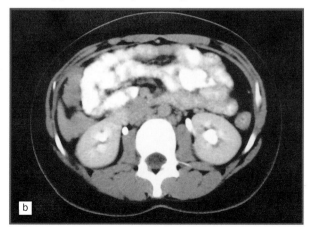

Figure 5.5 *Recurrent Hodgkin's disease affecting pelvic and para-aortic nodes (a), showing rapid response to second-line treatment with ChlVPP (b). The patient had received VEEP as primary chemotherapy.*

Table 5.3 Regimen for Stage IV Hodgkin's disease: OPPA × 2, COPP × 4 plus radiotherapy

Regimen	Drug dosage (mg/m²)	Drug administration on days
OPPA		
Vincristine	1.5	1, 8, 15
Procarbazine	100	1–15
Prednisolone	60	1–15
Adriamycin	40	1, 15
COPP		
Cyclophosphamide	500	1, 8
Vincristine	1.5	1, 8
Procarbazine	100	1–15
Prednisolone	40	1–15
Radiotherapy		
Involved nodes	20 Gy	
± lung and liver	12 Gy	
± bone	20–30 Gy	

Early relapses or those relapsing after initial advanced disease pose more of a problem. These will often have received multiagent hybrid regimens. A useful salvage regimen is EPIC (etoposide, prednisolone, ifosfamide and cisplatin) (Table 5.4) followed by extended-field irradiation and megatherapy.

What high-dose therapy should be used? There is little evidence that combination regimens are superior to high-dose melphalan alone. Combinations such as carmustine (BCNU), etoposide, AraC and melphalan

Table 5.4 EPIC regimen for relapsed Hodgkin's disease

Drug	Dose	Day of treatment					
		1	2	3	4	5	10
Etoposide	100 mg/m²	√	√	√	√		
Ifosfamide (+ mesna)	1 g/m²	√	√	√	√		
Prednisolone	60 mg/m²	√	√	√	√	√	
Cisplatin	60 mg/m²						√

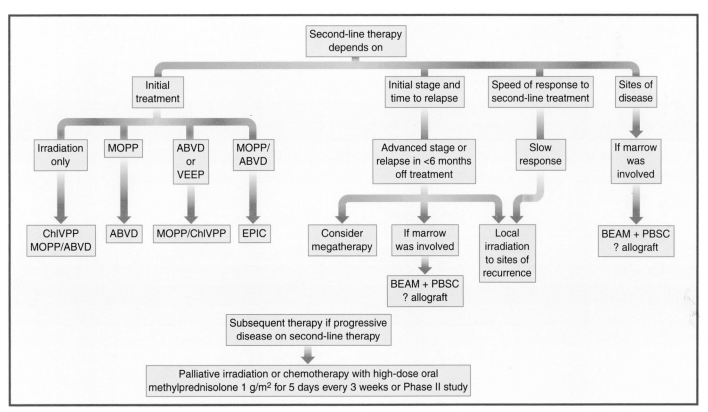

Figure 5.6 *Algorithm for treatment of relapsed Hodgkin's disease.*

are limited by the potential long-term toxicity of BCNU. Moreover, these patients will almost invariably have received prior etoposide and often cytarabine, and as the doses of these two drugs in BEAM are relatively low it is unlikely they add more than toxicity to the combination. The indications for high-dose therapy in Hodgkin's disease and the relative cost–benefit have been reviewed in adults, but the situation is much less clear in children. Because of the relative rarity of relapse in this condition, there is a need for multicentre collaboration to clarify the potential role of megatherapy in this disease. Broad guidelines for a treatment strategy for relapsed disease are given in Figure 5.6.

Further reading

Donaldson, S.S. and Link, M.P. (1987) Combined modality treatment with low dose radiation and MOPP chemotherapy for children with Hodgkin's disease. *Journal of Clinical Oncology* 5: 742–749.

Donaldson, S.S., Whitaker, S.J. Plowman, P.N. *et al.* (1990) Stage I–II pediatric Hodgkin's disease: long term follow-up demonstrates equivalent survival rates following different management schemes. *Journal of Clinical Oncology* 8: 1128–1137.

Ekert, H., Waters, K.D., Smith, P.J. *et al.* (1988) Treatment with MOPP or ChlVPP chemotherapy only for all stages of childhood Hodgkin's disease. *Journal of Clinical Oncology* 6: 1845–1850.

Fryer, C.J., Hutchinson, R.J., Krailo, M. *et al.* (1990) Efficacy and toxicity of 12 courses of ABVD chemotherapy followed by low dose regional radiation in advanced Hodgkin's disease in children: a report from the Children's Cancer Study Group. *Journal of Clinical Oncology* 8: 1971–1980.

Jones, R.J., Piantadosi, S., Mann, R.B. *et al.* (1990) Efficacy and toxicity of 12 courses of ABVD chemotherapy followed by low dose regional radiation in advanced Hodgkin's disease in children: a report from the Children's Cancer Study Group. *Journal of Clinical Oncology* 8: 527–539.

Leventhal, B.G. (1990) Management of Stage I–II Hodgkin's disease in children. *Journal of Clinical Oncology* 8: 1123–1124.

Oberlin, O., Leverger, G., Paquement, H. *et al.* (1992) Low-dose radiation therapy and reduced chemotherapy in childhood Hodgkin's disease. The experience of the French Society of Pediatric Oncology. *Journal of Clinical Oncology* 10: 1602–1608.

Radford, J.A., Cowan, R.A., Flanagan, M. *et al.* (1988) The significance of residual mediastinal abnormality on the chest radiograph following treatment for Hodgkin's disease. *Journal of Clinical Oncology* 6: 940–946.

Radford, M., Barrett, A., Martin, J. and Cotterill, S. (1991) Treatment of Hodgkin's disease in children. Study HDI. *Medical Pediatric Oncology* 19: 400.

Russell, K.R., Donaldson, S.S., Cox, R.S. and Kaplan, H.S. (1984) Childhood Hodgkin's disease: patterns of relapse. *Journal of Clinical Oncology* 2: 80–87.

Vecchi, V., Peleri, S., Burnelli, R. *et al.* (1993) Treatment of pediatric Hodgkin disease tailored to stage, mediastinal mass, and age. An Italian (AIEOP) multicentre study on 215 patients. *Cancer* 72: 2049–2057.

Wheeler, C., Antin, J.H. and Hallowell, A.W. (1990) Cyclophosphamide, carmustine and etoposide with autologous bone marrow transplantation in refractory Hodgkin's disease and non-Hodgkin's lymphoma: a dose-finding study. *Journal of Clinical Oncology* 8: 648–656.

PART II
Tumours of the central nervous system

CHAPTER 6

Low-grade astrocytomas

A. Michalski

Introduction

Primary malignancies of the central nervous system (CNS) constitute 20% of all childhood neoplasia. In the past, many texts referred to brain tumours as a relatively homogeneous group and large, historical series often presented the results of children treated in a standard manner but with little or no subdivision into histological subtype or location. Surgery was risky and many children were treated without a histopathological diagnosis. When tissue was obtained, histological diagnosis was based on a variety of different classifications with the use of many descriptive terms but relatively poor reproducibility. Before the advent of axial imaging (CT or MRI), localising tumours was based on clinical examination and crude, invasive tests such as pneumo-encephalography. Assessing the effectiveness of therapy was difficult as there was no way of radiologically determining response. Clinical assessment of response was complicated by the fact that patients often had had CSF diversion for hydrocephalus and had been started on steroids. It is, perhaps, not surprising that the development of rational, evidence-based therapy of CNS tumours has lagged so far behind that of other childhood tumours.

Currently, axial imaging allows accurate localisation of tumours as well as enabling us, in many cases at least, to gauge response. The improvement in surgical and anaesthetic techniques has meant that tumour tissue is obtainable from all but a few sites in the CNS with acceptable morbidity. The World Health Organization (WHO) classification has gained general acceptance, enabling pathologists to talk the same diagnostic language. However, problems with diagnosis and the assessment of response still exist and some of the key management difficulties are exemplified in the therapy of low-grade astrocytic tumours.

Low-grade astrocytomas comprise 45% of the tumours that arise in the CNS in childhood. The therapeutic challenges they pose are largely determined by their location and, operationally, tumours can be divided into:

- optic tract
- cerebellar
- cortical/supratentorial
- spinal cord
- brainstem.

Brainstem gliomas will be considered in a separate chapter. Before discussing each tumour site individually it will be instructive to define the pathology more clearly.

All classifications are arbitrary ways of grouping similar entities. Classifications are based on hypotheses of how tumours develop and will (indeed should) change as knowledge improves. The pathologist may want a classification that describes at what stage in the development of an astrocyte tumorigenesis occurred, but the clinician only wants the scheme to predict how the tumour will behave. In the WHO classification, low-grade astrocytomas are divided into pilocytic and fibrillary (which constitute the vast majority of paediatric tumours) but several other descriptive variants such as gemistocytic exist.

Pilocytic tumours are histologically less cellular and less diffuse than the fibrillary lesions. The older Kernohan classification graded astrocytomas numerically on their perceived 'aggressiveness' and grades I and II were low grade, grades III and IV high grade. The simple numerical nature of the classification did prompt some clinicians to treat grade II tumours more aggressively than grade I lesions, but, in reality, accurately distinguishing grades I and II was difficult. Individual astrocytomas are notoriously heterogeneous, with one area of the tumour looking quite different from another. Biopsies of lesions in difficult anatomical locations are often done stereotactically, and the small samples obtained increase the risk of sampling error. The edges of tumours often have a glial reaction and this can lead to an erroneous diagnosis of a low-grade astrocytoma. If the histology does not fit with the MRI scan or the clinical features, the possibility that the biopsy could be showing an 'edge' effect must be considered.

Optic tract tumours

Clinically, tumours of the optic tract can be divided into tumours of the optic nerve(s) not involving the chiasm and chiasmatic or hypothalamic lesions. Patients with neurofibromatosis (NF) type 1 are at increased risk of developing tumours but the risk is mainly for the optic nerve tumours. The true incidence of gliomas in the NF1 population is not known as published series are based on hospital populations, which are a selected group.

The natural history of optic tract tumours is very variable. Some lesions progress rapidly, resulting in loss of vision and hypothalamic disturbances, whereas others remain stable for many years with no therapy at all. Tumours can have periods of growth followed by spontaneous quiescence or even regression. The literature is divided, with some authors suggesting that these lesions are essentially hamartomatous (Imes and Hoyt, 1986) and should be left alone, whereas others recommend aggressive therapy (Pierce et al., 1990). The key issues are knowing whom to treat, what to treat with and when to stop; the rest is easy.

Who are the high-risk patients?

With chiasmatic tumours, young patients (under the age of 5 years and in particular under 1 year) appear to do worse, as do patients who are diagnosed with large tumours. For tumours of the optic nerve, the presence of NF1 appears to be associated with a more 'benign' outcome (Janss et al., 1995; Shuper et al., 1997). The decision of when to treat is also based on whether there is good clinical evidence of recent progression, so a 4-year-old patient with a chiasmatic tumour but stable vision over the last year would be a candidate for watching and waiting. If a small amount of tumour growth could potentially cause severe visual loss then treating early would be tempting. This is often the situation in a child with an optic nerve tumour that is involving the chiasm but with good visual function from the unaffected nerve, where growth of tumour into the chiasm could easily lead to blindness.

What should you treat with?

Unlike low-grade astrocytomas in other locations, attempts at primary resection of chiasmatic tumours are not recommended. That is not to say that surgery does not have a role. It is advisable (some would say mandatory) to biopsy large chiasmatic tumours as germinomas and gangliogliomas can mimic the radiological and clinical findings and need different therapy. Large cysts that are leading to symptoms should be aspirated and hydrocephalus treated appropriately. However, radical surgery to large chiasmatic or hypothalamic tumours virtually never achieves a total tumour clearance and often leads to permanent sequelae such as visual loss, diabetes insipidus and memory changes (especially when a trans-callosal route is used).

The inverse is true for tumours of the optic nerve. If vision in the affected nerve is reasonably good then a biopsy can be very hazardous and will contribute little useful information as the histology is nearly always predictable from the imaging. In a child with very poor vision but no chiasmatic involvement, resection of the tumour is curative.

A clear picture of the aims of therapy is very important in guiding choice of treatment. The definition of success is not a clear MRI scan but a functional child. If a residual mass remains at the end of therapy, one would not continue to add in different treatments as the mass may not change for very many years (if ever). The definition of response to treatment is different from that in any other tumour. Here, stable 'disease' is a perfectly respectable outcome.

The non-surgical therapies are chemotherapy and radiotherapy, and the choice between them is largely based on the age of the patient and the size of the tumour. Radiotherapy has more data to support its efficacy (especially with longer follow-up) (Cappelli *et al.*, 1998) but irradiating chiasmatic tumours in young children can result in serious side effects such as growth hormone deficiency, intellectual dysfunction and cerebrovascular disease. Chemotherapy is more morbid in the short term but has few, if any, late effects (Janss *et al.*, 1995; Shuper *et al.*, 1997). A variety of chemotherapy regimens have been used but there is now broad agreement that vincristine and carboplatin are the best initial choice (Packer *et al.*, 1993) and are used in the SIOP Low Grade Glioma Study for children 5 years of age or younger (Fig. 6.1). Stereotactically delivered fractionated radiotherapy is attractive in this setting, especially for older children with smaller tumours, but in most cases tumours will be too large for this approach and conventional radiotherapy will be delivered (the more focussed the better).

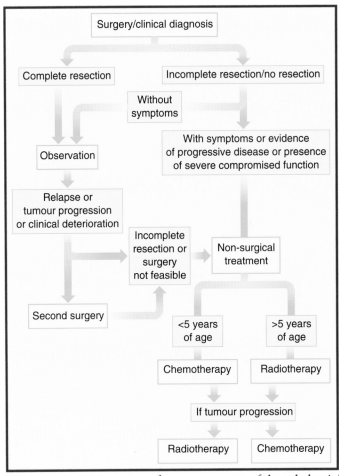

Figure 6.1 *SIOP strategy for management of hypothalamic/chiasmatic glioma and other low-grade glioma study.*

Clinical scenarios
Large hypothalamic chiasmatic tumour in an infant who is failing to thrive

Where a large hypothalamic chiasmatic tumour occurs in an infant who is failing to thrive, treatment should start without a watch-and-wait period as the tumour is almost bound to progress. The diencephalic syndrome with extreme wasting can occur and can co-exist with diabetes insipidus, visual loss and hydrocephalus. After biopsy and CSF diversion (if necessary), chemotherapy with vincristine and carboplatin should be commenced. If all goes well, the tumour will not grow and the patient will gain weight on nasogastric supplements, which can be tailed off over a number of months (Fig. 6.2).

Occasionally, rescanning at 10 weeks into therapy reveals tumour growth that can be associated with progression of symptoms, leading (on all usual oncological criteria) to therapy being stopped. However, the increase in the size of the tumour can

result from cyst formation (indicative of response). Figure 6.3 shows the increase in the size of a large tumour after 10 weeks of therapy during which the patient became blind and lost weight in spite of nasogastric feeds. Therapy was stopped but subsequent scans showed a delayed tumour response, which continued for 2 years. Therapy should not be stopped unless there is a greater than 25% increase in the area of the solid component (which is virtually impossible to measure with accuracy).

Although the tumour may be shrinking on scans, children can develop episodes of profound irritability (thought to be hypothalamic in origin) or even intermittent inappropriate secretion of antidiuretic hormone, so it is important not to assume that clinical 'deterioration' is caused by tumour growth.

The multifocal tumour

It is paradoxical that a tumour described as low grade can metastasise (Pollack *et al.*, 1994). Some patients

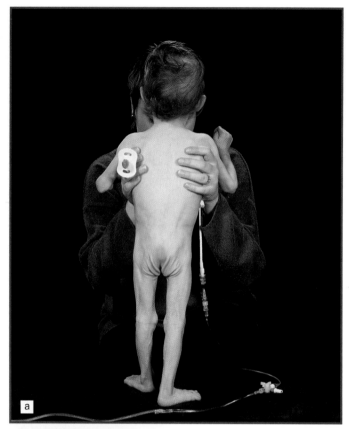

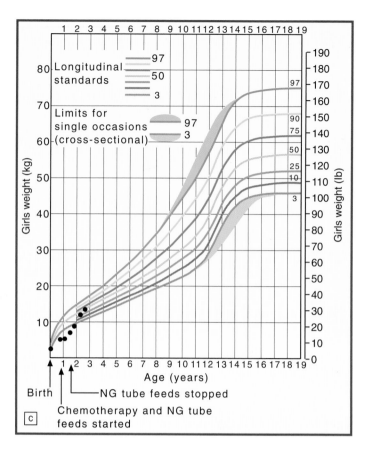

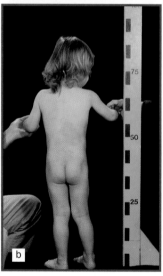

Figure 6.2 *A child (a) at diagnosis and (b) six months after completion of a year of vincristine and carboplatin chemotherapy. Her growth chart is also shown (c). Although the weight gain was dramatic, the tumour did not change in size over this period.*

have two or more discrete tumours with no leptomeningeal involvement and it is easy to be convinced that these are not metastatic, 'just' multifocal (Fig. 6.4). In other patients there is an identifiable primary tumour and leptomeningeal dissemination at diagnosis or (more uncommonly) at recurrence (Fig. 6.5). Even patients with widespread leptomeningeal involvement can be salvaged (with craniospinal radiation), but in the very young the late effects would be devastating. Multifocal disease is

controllable with chemotherapy alone in some patients.

The recurrent tumour

The survival of children with hypothalamic or chiasmatic astrocytomas is excellent (90% at 10 years) but in children presenting at 5 years of age or younger, the event-free survival is only 45%, indicating that these children are at risk of tumour growth and may require multiple therapeutic interventions. If chemotherapy was the initial treatment, radiotherapy should be instituted next unless the child is still very young, in which case second-line chemotherapy should be considered. There are few good data to guide in the choice of second-line therapy. Etoposide has been shown to be active in small series and has been given either as a daily oral dose or as intermittent infusions. With survival being so good, the increased risk of leukaemia with multiple-dose etoposide makes the daily oral schedule less attractive. Other therapies based on nitrosoureas have also been used (Prados *et al.*, 1997). Sadly, a proportion of children go on to have several recurrences with a step-wise loss of skills and function caused by both the tumour and the therapy.

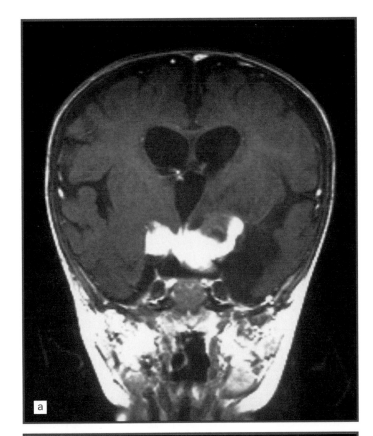

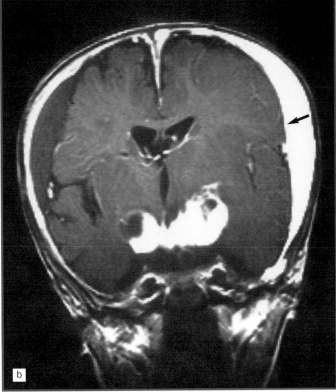

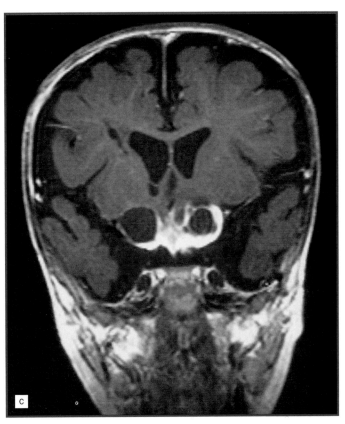

Figure 6.3 *(a) A saggital MR image of a patient with a proven low-grade astrocytoma. (b) After ten weeks of vincristine and carboplatin chemotherapy the tumour had grown in size but become more cystic. Note the subdural effusion (arrowed). (c) A saggital MR image of the same patient taken eight months after (b). The patient had received no further chemotherapy and yet the tumour had decreased in size.*

The unilateral optic nerve tumour

If the tumour is large and the vision in the eye is absent, then surgical removal of unilateral optic nerve

tumours is the treatment of choice as long as there is no chiasmatic involvement. The definition of chiasmatic involvement can be difficult and requires not only detailed MRI scans but the skills of a paediatric ophthalmologist. Visual acuity and fields are difficult to measure in young children, and there is increasing interest in the use of visual-evoked responses (VER) to measure postretinal dysfunction in a reproducible way (North *et al.*, 1994; Liu *et al.*, 1995). These electrical tests are not free from technical error and need to be performed by experts. Even in the best hands, the predictive value of a deteriorating VER in the absence of clinical or radiological evidence of chiasmatic involvement is uncertain. Similarly, a deteriorating VER in the absence of any other signs of tumour progression is not yet incontrovertible evidence for therapy to start. If there is residual vision in the affected eye, a watch-and-wait policy may be

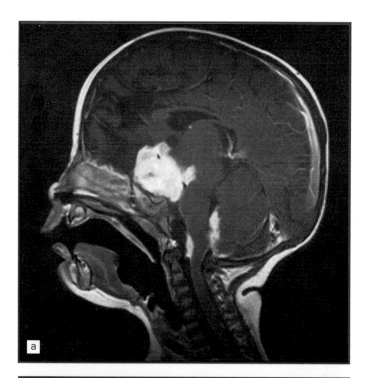

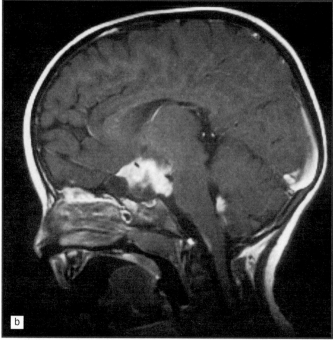

Figure 6.4 *A saggital MR image showing multifocal tumour deposits; a biopsy of the hypothalamic tumour showed a low-grade glioma (a). Three months after completion of a year of vincristine and carboplatin chemotherapy the tumour size was reduced (b).*

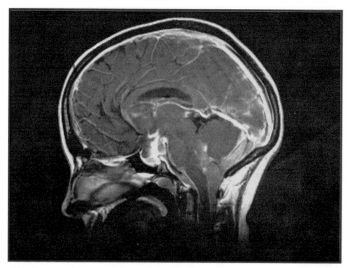

Figure 6.5 *A MR image showing leptomeningeal enhancement from a low-grade glioma.*

If the stump of the resected optic nerve is infiltrated by tumour, most clinicians would add chemotherapy but there are few data on this area. Definite chiasmatic involvement (on biopsy) should be treated with chemotherapy, which can cause a reduction in the size of the nerve tumour (Fig. 6.6).

Cerebellar astrocytomas

The cerebellum is the most common individual CNS structure to be affected with low-grade gliomas in childhood, and cerebellar astrocytomas form between 10 and 20% of all childhood CNS tumours. Neurosurgery is usually very successful as the sole therapeutic modality for cerebellar astrocytomas, and patients with completely resected tumour have a 90% long-term disease-free survival (Gajjar *et al.*, 1997). The tumours often have a significant cystic component and sometimes the solid part of the tumour is simply a small node in the cyst wall. The tumours can be large, with compression of the brain stem and surrounding structures. Compression is sometimes difficult to differentiate from invasion on MRI scanning, and careful clinical examination is often helpful; the presence of cranial nerve signs, hyper-reflexia or up-going plantar reflexes would be a concern. The therapy for residual disease after surgery is dependent on the age of the child and the presurgical clinical history. Large amounts of residual disease in a young child with a rapid clinical course are a much more worrying scenario than a slow progression of symptoms in an

adopted if there has not been a history of rapid change and especially if the patient has NF1. In the case of severely reduced vision secondary to a large tumour, battling with chemotherapy to save the residual vision is probably unjustified in young children as the eye is likely to become amblyopic.

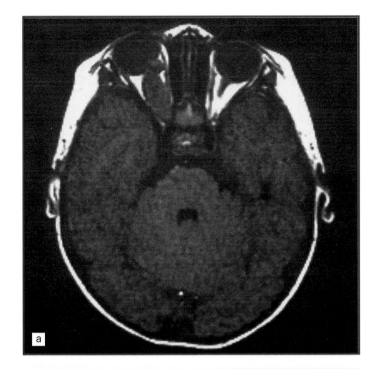

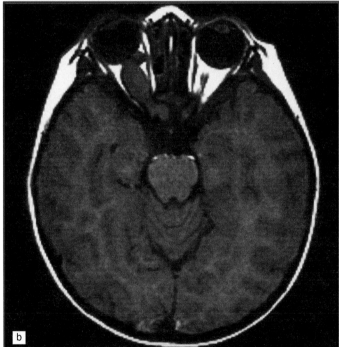

Figure 6.6 *MR images from a patient without NF1 who presented with an optic nerve tumour (a). After 30 weeks of therapy with vincristine and carboplatin the proptosis is reduced but the tumour has not shrunk markedly (b).*

older child with an almost complete resection. Many clinicians would watch and wait if there was residual disease, with the recommendation that further neurosurgery and adjunctive therapy (radiotherapy or chemotherapy) be used for recurrence. Some very large

tumours are not amenable to complete resection without causing significant neurological deficit. However, if the 'recurrence' is simply a re-filling of the cystic component without any change in the solid part of the tumour, drainage of the cyst alone can be tried in the first instance.

Cortical/supratentorial astrocytomas

The cortical or supratentorial tumours usually present as seizures with or without signs attributable to cortical dysfunction of the affected area (Fig. 6.7). A classical history would be of temporal lobe seizures (often misdiagnosed as behaviour disturbances or school problems) or an evolving hemiparesis with seizures. The tumours can be relatively large at diagnosis: sometimes surprisingly so compared with the paucity of clinical signs. The therapeutic dilemma that faces the clinicians is what to do with a neurologically functional child with a large tumour. In adult practice, the risk of malignant transformation of 'low-grade' tumours is said to be substantial, resulting in a firm belief that early, aggressive surgery is the way forward (Pollack *et al.*, 1995). In children, the risk of malignant transformation in an unresected tumour is low. The 'best' therapy is dependent

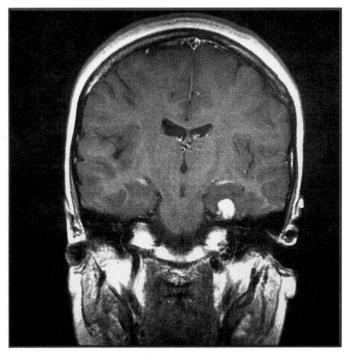

Figure 6.7 *A low-grade astrocytoma of the dominant temporal lobe presenting with seizures which were difficult to control.*

on individual circumstances, though neurosurgical resection should always be the first option. For example, if a neurologically intact child has a seizure a few months before major examinations at school and is found to have a cortical tumour, a biopsy followed by anticonvulsants with surgery delayed into an academically appropriate time for the child would be a good option. If a child stood to lose significant neurological function in an attempt at a complete resection, a biopsy followed by chemotherapy or radiotherapy would be a justifiable approach. Careful assessment of neuropsychological function before surgery is essential in some patients, and in a minority some form of 'cortical mapping' can accurately delineate what can be safely resected. Biopsies have to be of sufficient size to keep sampling error to a minimum.

Spinal cord tumours

Intramedullary spinal cord tumours comprise approximately 5% of all CNS tumours and two-thirds of these are astrocytomas, the vast majority of which are of low-grade histology. Any part of the spinal cord may be affected and over half the patients present with extensive tumours. The tumours grow slowly and the history often stretches over many months with recurrent visits to the medical services. Weakness, pain and sensory disturbances predominate, although sphincter problems can occur in lesions of the conus. Only 50% of the plain spinal radiographs are abnormal, which often leads to false reassurances being given to the families.

MRI is mandatory and lumbar punctures should not be attempted. The MRI scans usually show intramedullary tumour although occasionally 'mixed pictures' are seen in which both intra- and extramedullary disease is identified as shown in Figure 6.8. Surgery is the mainstay of therapy and in specialist units (who have both the equipment for intra-operative somato-sensory-evoked potential monitoring and the experience to use it) even large tumours can be near totally resected. For residual disease radiotherapy is the usual modality and in combination these therapies result in a 5-year survival of more than 70%.

Recurrences present therapeutic difficulties. If possible, surgical resection should be attempted again. There is anecdotal evidence that vincristine and carboplatin (as used for low-grade gliomas elsewhere in the CNS) can cause disease stabilisation. Sadly, some tumours continue to recur leading to progressive neurological deterioration and pain, which is often difficult to control. Patients with recurrences that involve the cervical spine are particularly difficult to

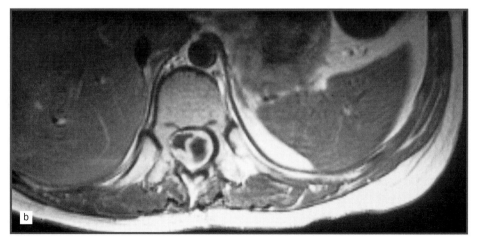

Figure 6.8 *Saggital (a) and axial (b) MR images of an extensive low-grade astrocytoma of the spinal cord with both intra- and extramedullary components.*

manage adequately. Here decreased respiratory function caused by paralysis has to be balanced with the need for strong opiate analgesia for intractable pain. The slow growth of the tumour in this situation is anything but a blessing.

Further reading

Cappelli, C., Grill, J., Raquin, M. *et al.* (1998) Long term follow up of 69 patients treated for optic pathway tumours before the chemotherapy era. *Archives of Disease in Childhood* 79: 334–338.

Gajjar, A., Sanford, R.A., Heindeman, R. *et al.* (1997) Low-grade astrocytoma: a decade of experience at St Jude Children's Research Hospital. *Journal of Clinical Oncology* 15: 2792–2799.

Imes, R.K. and Hoyt, W.F. (1986) Childhood chiasmal gliomas: update on the fate of patients in the 1969 San Francisco Study. *British Journal of Ophthalmology* 70: 179–182.

Janss, A.J., Grundy, R., Cnaan, A. *et al.* (1995) Optic pathway and hypothalamic/chiasmatic gliomas in children younger than 5 years with a 6 year follow-up. *Cancer* 75: 1051–1059.

Liu, G.T., Malloy, P., Needle, M. and Phillips, P. (1995) Optic gliomas in neurofibromatosis type 1: role of visual-evoked potentials. *Pediatric Neurology* 12: 89–90.

North, K., Cochineas, C., Tang, E. and Fagan, E. (1994) Optic gliomas in neurofibromatosis type 1: role of visual-evoked potentials. *Pediatric Neurology* 10: 117–123.

Packer, R.J., Langer, B., Ater, J. *et al.* (1993) Carboplatin and vincristine for recurrent and newly diagnosed low-grade gliomas of childhood. *Journal of Clinical Oncology* 11: 850–856.

Pierce, S.M., Barnes, P.D. Loeffler, J.S. *et al.* (1990) Definitive radiation therapy in the management of symptomatic patients with optic glioma: survival and long-term effects. *Cancer* 65: 45–52.

Pollack, I.F., Claassen, D., Al-Shboul, Q. *et al.* (1995) Low-grade gliomas of the cerebral hemispheres in children: an analysis of 71 cases. *Journal of Neurosurgery* 82: 536–547.

Pollack, I.F., Hurtt, M., Pang, D. and Leland Albright, A. (1994) Dissemination of low grade intracranial astrocytomas in children. *Cancer* 73: 2869–2878.

Prados, M.D., Edwards, M.S.B., Rabbitt, J. *et al.* (1997) Treatment of pediatric low-grade gliomas with a nitrosourea-based multiagent chemotherapy regimen. *Journal of Neuro-Oncology* 32: 235–241.

Shuper, A., Horev, G., Kornreich, L. *et al.* (1997) Visual pathway glioma: an erratic tumour with therapeutic dilemmas. *Archives of Disease in Childhood* 76: 259–263.

CHAPTER 7

Primitive neuro-ectodermal tumours of the CNS

A. Michalski

Introduction

Primitive neuro-ectodermal tumours (PNET) are the most contentious group of tumours within the CNS. After prolonged discussion, medulloblastoma (arising in the cerebellar vermis) was grouped together with other tumours that it resembled histologically and immunocytochemically even though there were identifiable differences in clinical behaviour and outcome. Ependymoblastoma is included in the PNET group; atypical rhabdoid/teratoid tumours are not. Even within the WHO classification, there are still differences among pathologists as to what does and what does not fit the diagnostic category. Even the nomenclature is confusing, as the letters PNET are also used for an entirely separate tumour outside the CNS (primitive peripheral neuro-ectodermal tumours are part of the spectrum of Ewing's sarcoma and many have the characteristic t(11;22) translocation). What is clear is that PNET of the CNS is not a single, homogeneous disease but rather a group of histologically similar conditions, and we should expect clinically distinct tumour types within this group. The challenge is identifying these groups at diagnosis and using this information to guide therapy.

Surgery and craniospinal radiotherapy with a boost to the site of the primary tumour have formed the basis of the therapy for PNET since the 1960s. The improvement in survival that has been evident during this time has resulted from the better use of these modalities. Even in recent trials, the single most common cause of recurrence was errors in the planning of the radiotherapy fields. In experienced centres, up to

70% of children with non-metastatic disease can be cured. However, the use of craniospinal radiation in young children is associated with profound neuropsychological and endocrine sequelae. The younger the child, the more profound the sequelae. There has been an understandable desire to reduce the sequelae without compromising cure and the use of chemotherapy has been central to this issue. There is immense controversy about the use of chemotherapy and radiotherapy and the following clinical scenarios will illustrate a personal view of the issues.

Who are the high-risk patients?

Certain risk factors are generally accepted. Children with imageable metastatic disease or with subtotal resections fare poorly. It is uncertain how much residual disease is needed to confer a worse prognosis. Some groups define residual disease as more than 1.5 cm^3 (which is difficult to measure with precision), whereas in other centres any radiologically evident tumour counts as 'residual'. Some children have clear MRI scans but the neurosurgeon reports that there was invasion of the floor of the fourth ventricle that was not amenable to resection; we do not know if this 'subradiographic' disease is an adverse prognostic factor. The prognostic significance of other factors is even less certain. The presence of malignant cells in the CSF is classified as M1 disease, but there are relatively loose criteria for this diagnosis. When was the CSF taken: at surgery before disturbance of the tumour, or after surgery, and if so how long after and from which site? Do isolated malignant cells count or is it clumps of cells? Is it morphology or immunostaining or both that count? There is some published evidence (largely in the form of abstracts rather than peer-reviewed journals) to suggest that M1 disease is an adverse factor, but considerably more discipline in definition and reporting is necessary before this can be accepted.

Age is another complicated prognostic variable. Children under 3 years of age have fared worse, but the reasons for this are not completely clear. Certainly, some groups have found that young children have higher-risk disease with less complete resections and more metastatic disease. The use of craniospinal radiotherapy and the doses administered are much more variable in the very young, as the late effects are so profound. Whether these two variables alone are enough to explain the poor results in the under 3-year-old age group is uncertain; it may be that young children have biologically more aggressive disease in a way that formal staging criteria and histology are unable to determine.

Extrapolating from the advances in neuroblastoma and rhabdomyosarcoma management, one could postulate that changes at the molecular level could be used as prognostic variables. Currently, loss of heterozygosity for chromosome 17 has been postulated as being a predictor of bad outcome, and other molecular 'fingerprints' (such as amplification of the oncogene c-myc or co-expression of two members of the epidermal growth factor receptor family, ErbB-2 and ErbB-4) have also been suggested.

Site is another prognostic factor as supratentorial PNET have a worse outcome than the classical 'medulloblastoma' arising in the posterior fossa. The factors indicating prognosis are shown in Box 7.1.

Box 7.1 Adverse prognostic factors in CNS PNET

Definite factors:
  Metastatic disease
  Residual local disease
  Young age
  Supratentorial location
Probable factors:
  M1 disease (cells in CSF with a clear MRI scan)
  Loss of heterozygosity for chromosome 17
  Oncogene amplification
  Co-expression of ErbB-2 and ErbB-4

The standard-risk patient more than 3 years of age: what is the best treatment?

In children with no evidence of metastatic disease, there is no randomised trial that shows the addition of chemotherapy to surgery and craniospinal radiotherapy is of benefit (Evans *et al.*, 1990; Tait *et al.*, 1990). However, many units regard the use of chemotherapy in PNET as proven. Certainly, there is no doubt that PNET is a chemoresponsive tumour, with response rates of up to 70% with agents such as the platinums (often in combination with etoposide), cyclophosphamide and other alkylating agents. Individual centres have published 5-year survival rates of 85% (Packer *et al.*, 1994) which are interesting but not conclusive proof that chemotherapy gives a survival advantage to a more unselected population of patients.

There is a difference in intent between different protocols:

- to increase cure when used with full-dose neuraxis irradiation
- to delay radiotherapy
- to reduce dose of neuraxis radiation
- to allow radiotherapy to be omitted completely.

Some protocols are designed to improve survival by adding chemotherapy to full-dose craniospinal radiation (Kuhl *et al.*, 1993). Others aim to reduce the dose of craniospinal radiation in order to inflict less neurocognitive damage on the survivors. It is still uncertain what the lowest effective dose of craniospinal radiation when used as sole therapy actually is. Traditionally, 36 Gy has been given to the craniospinal axis but there is some evidence to suggest that lower doses, even as low as 24 Gy, may be as effective. Chemotherapy has been used to try to reduce the dose of radiation and keep the survival the same. Goldwein used chemotherapy with a neuraxis radiotherapy dose as low as 1800 cGy with an actuarial survival of 69% at 4 years (Goldwein *et al.*, 1993). An attempt at using chemotherapy to omit 'prophylactic' cranial radiation entirely (i.e. surgery followed by chemotherapy, then radiotherapy to the tumour bed and to the spine but not the brain, followed by further chemotherapy) was unsuccessful as 9 of the 13 patients relapsed in the group with un-irradiated brains (Bouffet *et al.*, 1992). One pilot study is investigating the use of chemotherapy before surgery (patients are initially treated with a biopsy and a CSF diversion procedure without an attempt at resection) to try and shrink the tumour and allow for more complete surgical resection.

The use of chemotherapy has its problems. If given after craniospinal irradiation, the dose intensity has to be low as myelosuppression is a problem. If given before radiotherapy, the chemotherapy doses can be higher but there will inevitably be a delay in the administration of radiotherapy, which remains the single most active agent in PNET. Chemotherapy given concurrently with irradiation with growth factor support is being investigated but is certainly not routine. In truth, we do not really know if chemotherapy adds to survival and have to ask the question in the context of randomised trials if the answer is ever to be known.

High-risk patients more than 3 years of age at diagnosis

There are two groups of high-risk patients over 3 years of age: those with residual local disease and those with metastatic disease. In children with residual local disease, it is generally accepted that second-look surgery should be given careful consideration. Sometimes brain that has been compressed by a large tumour 'relaxes' back into the space created by the resection and allows easier surgery on what was previously inaccessible tumour. The use of chemotherapy is still contentious here. However, many groups give pre-radiotherapy chemotherapy using active but myelosuppressive agents such as carboplatin, etoposide and cyclophosphamide. Other units given radiotherapy first and follow on with the 'Packer' regimen of cisplatin, vincristine and lomustine (CCNU), which is less myelosuppressive but can cause ototoxicity or nephropathy.

Metastases in PNET are nearly always confined to the CNS and less than 1% of patients have disease outside the CNS at diagnosis. Within the CNS the pattern of metastatic disease is variable, with some children presenting with diffuse leptomeningeal

enhancement on MRI scanning whereas others have lumps of localised disease. It appears that the former pattern is associated with the poorer outcome. As leptomeningeal enhancement can occur after neurosurgery and persist for months, it is imperative to perform an MRI of the spine before surgery to stage the CNS accurately.

Around 40% of patients with metastatic disease have been reported as being cured with surgery and radiotherapy, and irradiation certainly produces some dramatic resolutions of disease (Fig. 7.1). Most units would use chemotherapy to try to improve the chances of cure. The use of cisplatin, CCNU and vincristine after radiotherapy has been reported as giving a 5-year progression-free survival of 67% (Packer *et al.*, 1994). If the child has symptoms from the disseminated disease, especially spinal cord compression, then radiotherapy should be given first (before chemotherapy) as this modality not only stands the best chance of being effective but probably works more

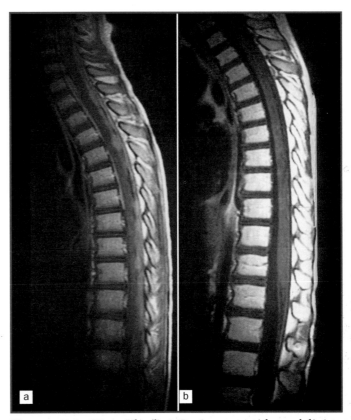

Figure 7.1 *T1-weighted MR images with gadolinium enhancement from a patient with diffuse leptomeningeal dissemination of PNET before (a) and 6 weeks after radiotherapy (b) showing clearance of disease. Note that in (b) the black signal of CSF now surrounds the spinal cord whereas in (a) there was tumour signal around the cord.*

quickly. The use of high-dose chemotherapy has increased recently for patients with high-risk disease. Cytoreduction with standard chemotherapy followed by a high-dose procedure with autologous rescue (with stem cells) has been tried but does delay the administration of radiotherapy, perhaps inappropriately. Again, we are only going to learn the best way of managing these children if we collect cooperative data in well-constructed trials.

Children under the age of 3 years

Irradiating the developing brain gives rise to profound neuropsychological and endocrine sequelae. Children who have received whole brain irradiation at under 3 years of age have decreased intelligence quotients (IQs), which may continue to deteriorate with age. Their school performance is even worse than their decreased IQ would predict because of difficulties with concentration and attention. They are unlikely to be employable and their social relationships may be poor (Kiltie et al., 1997). It is important to realise that there is no 'safe' age for radiotherapy, but the younger the child is when they are irradiated the more profound the sequelae. Operationally, many groups use the age of 3 years as a cut off, but others would omit or reduce the dose of radiotherapy up to 5 years of age.

These difficulties have led to interest in the use of chemotherapy. The intent of the original protocols was to delay radiotherapy, which was then given to all patients at full dose; later protocols aimed to delay radiotherapy and reduce the dose to the neuraxis in those with a good response to chemotherapy (Duffner et al., 1993). Further studies then omitted neuraxis irradiation altogether and some aimed to avoid all radiotherapy in primary treatment (Lashford et al., 1996). The chemotherapy protocols were initially given over a long period of time (until the child was 3 years of age) and so were not very dose intensive. The median time to recurrence was only 6 months, the relapsing children were still very young and many did not receive radiotherapy even at recurrence.

Some success was reported with these strategies but in most series the event-free survival was poor. There is some evidence that risk groups exist and young children with metastatic disease present the greatest

challenge. For high-risk patients, current strategies include the use of conventional chemotherapy for cytoreduction followed by high-dose chemotherapy with autologous stem cell rescue instead of neuraxis radiation. Other groups are piloting multiple high-dose procedures with autologous haematological support and growth factors. Again, trials of therapy are mandatory if we are to learn how best to treat this challenging group of patients.

The relapsed patient

There are three main groups of relapsed patients:

1. Patients who have not received radiotherapy as part of their initial therapy.
2. Patients who have been irradiated and now have local or purely focal recurrences.
3. Patients who have been irradiated and now have metastatic recurrences.

Group 1
Maximal surgical resection and radiotherapy can salvage a high proportion of the children who have not received initial therapy that included radiotherapy. If the child is still very young, high-dose chemotherapy procedures can be attempted, as in groups 2 and 3.

Group 2
Some evidence is now available that suggests that some of the children who have been irradiated and who only have local/focal recurrences can be salvaged with aggressive surgery and high-dose chemotherapy with autologous stem cell rescue (Graham et al., 1997; Dunkel et al., 1998). It is probably not worth considering high-dose chemotherapy in the presence of substantial residual disease. There is no best bet for high-dose therapy and the toxicity of many of the regimens is serious, with an appreciable toxic mortality.

Group 3
There is only anecdotal evidence of cure in children who have been irradiated and have metastatic recurrence. Therapy is experimental, and serious consideration should be given to other approaches, such as oral etoposide, that can slow disease

progression or even give rise to partial remissions and can provide very good symptom relief. The risk of late leukaemia from etoposide is not relevant for this population. Trials of phase 1 and 2 agents can be offered to children, but the families need to be aware that these do not realistically hold out chances of cure. Patterns of metastatic disease vary; some patients have aggressive leptomeningeal dissemination (Fig. 7.2) whereas others can go many months with slow progression of a few isolated deposits (Fig. 7.3).

Before the advent of salvage therapies, the mean time from recurrence to death was only 5 months (Torres *et al.*, 1994). Not all patients will be in a fit enough neurological state to undergo intensive chemotherapy and not all families will want their children to spend a large part of what may be only a short survival having aggressive therapy. Oral etoposide (50 mg/m^2 per day for 21 days followed by 7 days off therapy) can be useful in slowing disease progression. Other families will want to participate in phase 1 and 2 trials of new agents. What must not be forgotten is that some families will be keen on good symptom control alone, to allow the children to spend as much time as possible at home. There is no single 'medically right' answer and it is vital to have frank and open discussions with the families and the children to select the most appropriate way forward.

Follow-up of children treated for PNET

There are two main reasons to follow up children with PNET. Firstly, all children will need some degree of input to maximise their function after therapy. Those treated with radiotherapy will need assessment of growth and development by an endocrinologist. Most will need growth hormone therapy. The tumour and surgery may have left the children with significant neurological dysfunction, for which physiotherapy, occupational therapy and mobility aids may be necessary. Radiotherapy will have created some neuropsychological problems and accurate assessment of these difficulties is mandatory as it allows the provision of extra educational help. It is uncertain how much of the problems are amenable to extra tuition, but simply allowing children to fail educationally is not a defensible option.

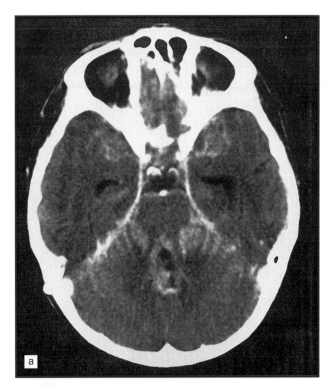

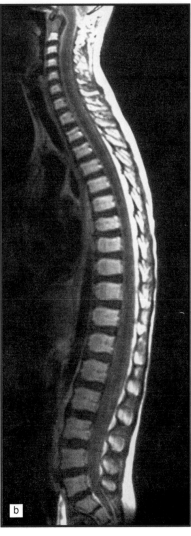

Figure 7.2 *CT scan (a) and MR image (b) showing diffuse leptomeningeal disease in a child with PNET.*

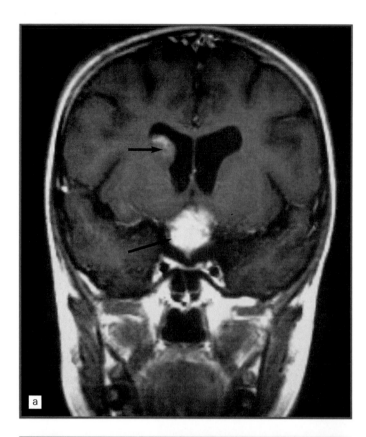

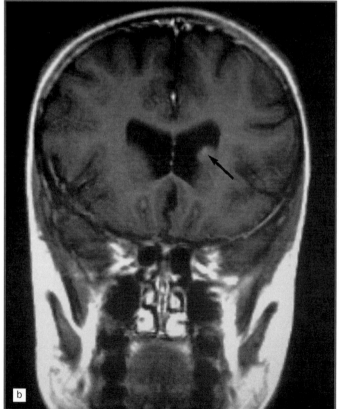

Figure 7.3 *(a,b) Coronal MR images showing multifocal recurrent disease in a child treated for a medulloblastoma with surgery and craniospinal radiotherapy. These three sites of disease (arrowed) progressed slowly over 3 years.*

Secondly, we should look for recurrence of the disease, especially as a proportion of children who do have recurrent disease can be cured. It is uncertain how best this can be achieved, though a careful history and clinical examination are mandatory. The value of routine MRI scanning has been questioned, as children who have a normal MRI scan can show recurrence symptomatically a couple of months later (Torres *et al.*, 1994). Scanning any more frequently than 3-monthly places an unacceptable burden of worry on the families and is hugely expensive. Most units still scan routinely if only to document the event-free survival of current therapy. A check list for follow-up is shown in Box 7.2.

Conclusion

After two decades of the use of chemotherapy, there are still more questions than answers in the therapy of PNET. Unless patients are entered into trials, we will remain ignorant about the optimal way to treat this heterogeneous group of patients.

Box 7.2 Check list for follow-up of PNET

Has the child relapsed?
- history and neurological examination
- role of surveillance scanning unclear

Neuropsychological problems
- developmentally appropriate neuropsychometric test
- school performance
- mood, relationships

Endocrine problems
- weigh, measure and plot on charts
- pubertal status
- measurement of growth hormone, T4, TSH, gonadotrophins (with endocrinologist's support)

Physical problems
- ataxia
- long tract signs
- nutrition
- seizures
- vision/hearing

Further reading

Bouffet, E., Bernard, J.L., Frappaz, D. *et al.* (1992) M4 protocol for cerebellar medulloblastoma: supratentorial radiotherapy may not be avoided. *International Journal of Radiation Oncology, Biology and Physics* 24: 79–85.

Duffner, P.K., Horowitz, M.E., Krischer, J.P. *et al.* (1993) Post operative chemotherapy and delayed radiation in children less than three years of age with malignant brain tumors. *New England Journal of Medicine* 328: 1725–1731.

Dunkel, I.J., Boyett, J.M., Yates, A. *et al.* (1988) High dose carboplatin thiotepa and etoposide with autologous stem-cell rescue for patients with recurrent medulloblastoma. *Journal of Clinical Oncology* 16: 222–228.

Evans, A.E., Jenkin, D.T., Sposto, R. *et al.* (1990) The treatment of medulloblastoma: results of a prospective randomised trial of radiation therapy with and without CCNU, vincristine and prednisolone. *Journal of Neurosurgery* 72: 572–582.

Goldwein, J.W., Radcliffe, J., Packer, R.J. *et al.* (1993) Results of a pilot study of low-dose craniospinal radiation therapy plus chemotherapy for children younger than 5 years with primitive neuroectodermal tumours. *Cancer* 71: 2647–2652.

Graham, M.L., Herndon, J.E., Casey, J.R., *et al.* (1997) High dose chemotherapy with autologous stem cell rescue in patients with recurrent and high-risk pediatric brain tumors. *Journal of Clinical Oncology* 15: 1814–1823.

Kiltie, A.E., Lashford, L.S. and Gattamaneni, H.R. (1997) Survival and late effects in medulloblastoma patients treated with craniospinal irradiation under three years old. *Medical and Pediatric Oncology* 28: 348–354.

Kuhl, J., Berthold, F., Bode, U. *et al.* (1993) Preradiation chemotherapy of children with poor-prognosis medulloblastoma: response rate and toxicity of the ifosfamide-containing multidrug regimen HIT "88/'89'. *American Journal of Pediatric Hematology/Oncology* 15 (Suppl. A): S67–S71.

Lashford, L.S., Campbell, R.H.A., Gattamaneni, H.R. *et al.* (1996) An intensive multiagent chemotherapy regimen for brain tumours occurring in very young children. *Archives of Disease in Childhood* 74: 219–223.

Packer, R.J., Sutton, L.N., Elterman, R. *et al.* (1994) Outcome for children with medulloblastoma treated with radiation and cisplatin, CCNU and vincristine chemotherapy. *Journal of Neurosurgery* 81: 690–698.

Tait, D.M., Thornton-Jones, H., Bloom, H.J. *et al.* (1990) Adjuvant chemotherapy for medulloblastoma: the first multicentre controlled trial of the International Society of Pediatric Oncology (SIOP 1). *European Journal of Cancer* 26: 464–469.

Torres, C.F., Rebsamen, S., Silber, J.H. *et al.* (1994) Surveillance scanning of children with medulloblastoma. *New England Journal of Medicine* 330: 892–895.

CHAPTER 8
High-grade and brainstem glioma

A. Michalski

Introduction

Prognostically this will be the most depressing chapter in the book. The inclusion of both these diseases in a chapter of their own rather than as part of an 'other' section is because the management of disease with a poor prognosis is difficult. At diagnosis, the therapeutic dilemma is offering best known therapy, which has a very poor but not zero chance of cure, versus offering the novel and the experimental; at recurrence, whether to offer phase 1 and 2 trials versus good palliative care. When the illness is terminal the change of intent moves to work towards a dignified and symptom-free remainder of life and inevitable death. Sadly, with current therapy, most of our patients with brainstem tumours or high-grade gliomas will die of their disease. The management of poor-prognosis and terminal illness is not optional.

High-grade glioma

The diagnosis of a high-grade glial tumour is often suspected on the 'diagnostic' MR image. A solid tumour with considerable signal change around it, especially on T2-weighted MR images, is often seen (Fig. 8.1). However, even MR imaging cannot easily define the full extent of the tumour. Although the contrast-enhancing area on MR images is found to be 'solid' tumour, stereotactic biopsies taken at the limits of the T2 signal show tumour cells infiltrating normal brain.

Clearly, a 'complete resection' as judged as the removal of the contrast-enhancing lesion still leaves a

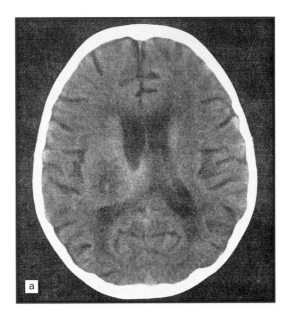

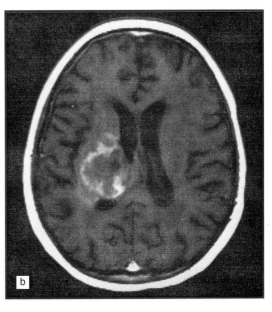

Figure 8.1 *The typical appearances of a glioblastoma multiforme. (a) CT scan; (b) MR image.*

considerable amount of tumour behind. However, even having said that a truly complete resection of a high-grade glial tumour is almost never performed, the extent of surgical resection remains one of the most powerful predictors of outcome (Finlay *et al.*, 1995; Sposto *et al.*, 1989). As the 'completely resected' tumours tend to be cortical and those for which resection is incomplete are deep, thalamic; it may be that the biology of tumours in these two sites differs. It could be, therefore, a difference in disease biology and not the degree of resection that is responsible for the differences in survival that are observed between the two groups. Should surgical resections be even more aggressive; accepting permanent neurological sequelae as the only way to cure? There is little evidence that even more aggressive surgery will increase the chances of a truly complete resection for most patients as it is likely that some residual disease will still be left. Our neurosurgical practice is to attempt maximum resection (using neuro-navigation if necessary) but to steer away from surgery that would inevitably cause neurological damage.

The histopathology of the tumour affects outcome, with glioblastoma multiforme faring worse than anaplastic astrocytoma, which in turn fares worse than 'other' forms of high-grade glioma (Finlay *et al.*, 1995; Sposto *et al.*, 1989). However, it has to be recognised that the histopathological subclassification of high-grade glial tumours is difficult, and even experienced neuropathologists may differ on individual cases. Interpretation of the results of therapy in series without central or independent pathological review should be done with caution. Our current understanding of the factors affecting prognosis in high-grade glioma is shown in Box 8.1.

The key therapeutic issue is how to deal with the residual disease that almost always remains after surgery. Radiotherapy certainly causes tumours to shrink and does improve neurological state. Sadly,

---

Box 8.1 Factors denoting poor prognosis in childhood high-grade glioma

Non-cortical location (e.g. thalamus)

Incomplete resection

Glioblastoma multiforme on histology

Older age

---

these responses are often shortlived and the majority of patients relapse within a short time frame. Increasing the effect of radiotherapy has been the subject of much work. In adults, increasing the total dose delivered to the tumour from around 50 Gy to 75 Gy has not resulted in an increase in long-term survival, though there were modest improvements as the dose of radiation increased (Salazar *et al.*, 1979). At doses above 70 Gy the incidence of radionecrosis increases. Depressingly, many radiation oncologists have concluded that the radiosensitivity of high-grade glial tumours is the same as that of normal brain and that there is, therefore, no therapeutic index to exploit. If one cannot increase the dose then why not restrict the radiation field? The problem is that infiltrating tumour cells can be found over 3 cm from the main tumour mass and too restricted a radiation field will result in relapses at the edges of the field. Tumour infiltration also restricts the potential utility of many of the novel therapies that have been tried, such as photodynamic therapy (with light sources implanted during the neurosurgical resection), intracavity carmustine, herpes virus delivery followed by ganciclovir, and others. All of these agents may theoretically allow tumour cell kill, some claim specificity for growing tumour but currently none can penetrate far enough into brain parenchyma to seek out the edge of tumour infiltration (Kadota, 1996). Making the tumour more sensitive to radiotherapy has also been investigated using hyperbaric oxygen or agents such as halogenated pyrimidines, but this has not, as yet, been sufficiently successful to be integrated into standard practice (Rodriguez and Kinsella, 1991).

The role of chemotherapy is hotly disputed. Most countries have chemotherapy protocols that are intended to delay or avoid radiotherapy for patients under 3 years of age at diagnosis (Duffner *et al.*, 1993). Very young children with high-grade gliomas do appear to have a better prognosis than older children, who, in turn, fare better than adults (Phuphanich *et al.*, 1984).

For patients over the age of 3 years at diagnosis, the only randomised trial of the use of chemotherapy following surgery and radiotherapy did appear to show some benefit for the use of lomustine and vincristine, but subsequent subgroup analysis suggested this may have been restricted to children with glioblastoma multiforme (Sposto *et al.*, 1989). Hence, lomustine and vincristine dual therapy is regarded in some centres as 'standard' therapy; however, with a 5-year survival of 42% at best (Sposto *et al.*, 1989) (and a progression-free survival of 16% at 5 years in a more recent study by Finlay *et al.*, 1995) it must be seen as a 'bronze' standard rather than a 'gold' standard. The continued use of lomustine and vincristine outside of a clinical trial actually prevents the acquisition of data on what may be the effective agents. In the UK, relatively few patients who relapse with high-grade gliomas are enrolled on phase 2 clinical trials. In a condition with such a poor survival it is, in the author's opinion, ethical and necessary to use a phase 2 window model where individual chemotherapy agents are tested at a maximum tolerated dose in patients with residual disease after surgery. If there is a response, the agent is continued after radiotherapy; if not or in patients with no residual disease standard therapy continues (see Figure 8.2).

High-dose chemotherapy has its advocates, but although responses have been reported (McCowage *et al.*, 1998), its use has to be seen as experimental (Mason *et al.*, 1998). Oligodendrogliomas are rare in

children but are a subgroup in which chemotherapy has a definite role (Cairncross *et al.*, 1994).

Sadly, the majority of children with high-grade glial tumours will have a relapse of their disease. In only a small minority will the recurrence be amenable to a second curative attempt. The discussion about trials of investigational agents versus good symptom care need time, understanding and empathy. The survival time from recurrence is often short and many families do not want to spend what little time they have with their child in hospital being worked up for phase 1 or 2 trials. Conversely, the availability of an investigational agent programme allows those families who want to 'try everything' to remain in the hands of the team they have known throughout their child's care. Discussions about good symptom care are essential (see below).

Brainstem gliomas

There are three broad clinical scenarios encompassed by this term and each relates to an anatomical location within the brainstem.

The midbrain tumour

Tumours arising in the upper midbrain or tectum, such as the example shown in Figure 8.3, may present with

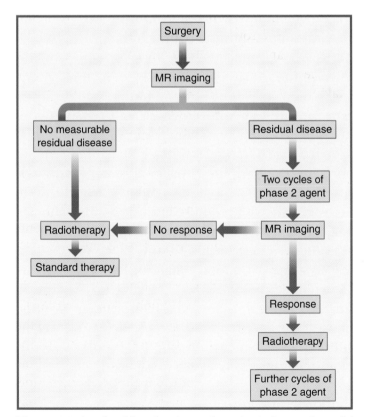

Figure 8.2 *An algorithm showing a phase 2 window study model that could be used to find active agents in high-grade glioma.*

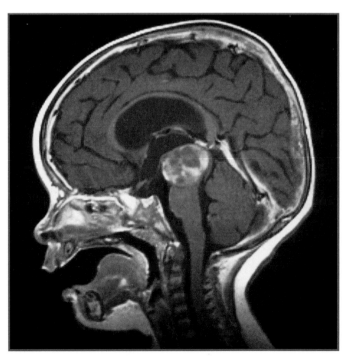

Figure 8.3 *A MR image of an unusually bulky tectal plate lesion, causing failure of upgaze and hydrocephalus.*

hydrocephalus without any other signs, though involvement of the tectal plate can lead to failure of up-gaze. It is likely that many children previously diagnosed as having idiopathic hydrocephalus have had these tumours and, even though they have been treated with CSF diversion procedures alone, these patients have not had tumour progression (Boydston *et al.*, 1991).

The pontine tumour

The pontine tumour is, numerically, by far the most common type of brainstem tumour and has an appalling prognosis. Classically, these lesions are diffuse infiltrating tumours that expand the pons, as shown in Figure 8.4. They often do not enhance on MR images and are hypodense on CT scans. The children present with short histories of multiple cranial nerve signs and long tract involvement. There may be changes in mood or affect. Hydrocephalus is uncommon. The median survival is 9–12 months and over 90% of patients are dead 18 months from diagnosis.

The cervicomedullary tumour

Tumours that arise in the cervical/medullary region have two distinct patterns of clinical presentation: spinal cord dysfunction or defects in the lower cranial

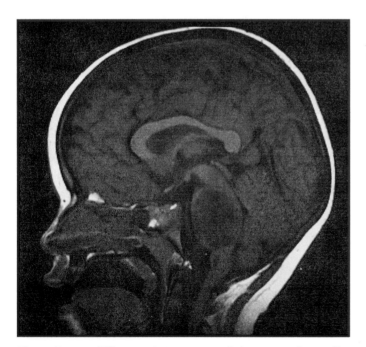

Figure 8.4 *A diffuse intrinsic pontine glioma. Note the swollen pons and the lack of contrast enhancement on this T1-weighted gadolinium-enhanced study.*

nerves. Spinal cord problems include neck pain and long tract signs, with cranial nerve dysfunction occurring late if at all. The second group presents with difficulty swallowing, changes in the character of speech, followed later by upper motor neuron signs. In both groups, the duration of symptoms can be long (over a year) and the majority of tumours are either low-grade gliomas or gangliogliomas, though ependymomas and the occasional high-grade glioma can occur. Radical resection of the low-grade tumours can result in neurological recovery and long-term survival but carries risks of devastating neurological complications.

What is the role of surgery?

In the tectal tumours, CSF diversion is the only surgical intervention that is needed in the first instance. If possible, third ventriculostomy may be preferable to ventriculo-peritoneal shunting as it obviates the risks of implanted tubing in a life-long condition. Only if the tumour grows as observed on MR imaging would the author recommend tumour biopsy. In dorsally exophytic tumours of the cervicomedullary junction, an attempt at radical removal should be made but only by experienced paediatric neurosurgeons. For the classical diffuse intrinsic pontine tumours the author does not recommend even a biopsy. Any surgical intervention carries a finite risk of complications (around 10% in most series) and the histology does not correlate well with prognosis and certainly does not direct therapy. The majority of children who have been reported as having low-grade glial tumours of the pons are dead within 2 years. This is perhaps not surprising as histologically there is considerable heterogeneity within diffuse intrinsic pontine gliomas and the necessity to take small biopsies will lead to sampling error occurring. Clearly, if the findings on scans are atypical, a focal enhancing lesion in the pons for example, a biopsy will be necessary. Primitive neuroectodermal tumours can present as pontine masses and need very different therapy. A recent consensus statement on the role of surgery in brainstem tumours is shown in Table 8.1.

Radiotherapy issues

In children with progressive midbrain tumours or in patients with tumours of the cervicomedullary

Table 8.1 The role of surgery in the management of brainstem tumours

Site	Likely pathology	Surgical management[1]
Midbrain		
Tectal plate	Low-grade astrocytoma	Observe (CSF diversion as necessary)
Other	As for pons	
Pons		
Diffuse	High-grade astrocytoma	Biopsy not recommended; proceed to radiotherapy (± chemotherapy)
Cystic	Low- or high-grade astrocytoma	Drain cyst; debulk solid component
Exophytic	Low- or high-grade astrocytoma	Debulk
Focal intrinsic	Low- or high-grade astrocytoma	Debulk or radiotherapy (dependent on position and neurological deficit)
Medulla	As for pontine	Neurological results of radical surgery poor
Cervico-medullary	Low-grade astrocytoma	Radical removal

[1] When diagnosis is in doubt then a biopsy of any lesion should be considered. All cases should be assessed and treated under the auspices of an established paediatric neuro-oncology team.

Courtesy of Mr Richard Hayward, Consultant Neurosurgeon, Great Ormond St Hospital for Children, London.

junction in whom surgery has been incomplete, radiotherapy can be curative. In both of the above clinical conditions, chemotherapy in the form of vincristine and carboplatin may be used as primary treatment in children less than 5 years of age or in those patients whose tumours recur after radiation therapy. The schedule is that employed for low-grade gliomas in other locations.

In infiltrative pontine gliomas, radiotherapy is the only therapy that alters the clinical course of the disease, leading to symptomatic improvement but not cure. In order to try to increase the effectiveness of radiotherapy, the tumour dose has been increased to 70 Gy using schedules of hyperfractionation to keep the biological equivalent dose to normal tissue the same as in more conventional schedules, which deliver 54 Gy. However, survival was not improved and local

tumour swelling during radiation was increased, with a concomitant increase in steroid dependency. In the small number of patients who did survive their disease, there was an increased incidence of vasculopathy. Hence, most units now use a total tumour dose of 54 Gy delivered conventionally in 1.8 Gy fractions daily. Even with this fractionation regimen, some children experience neurological deterioration during radiotherapy. Careful observation, especially of bulbar function, is necessary during the course of radiotherapy; if deterioration occurs, steroids can be effective.

Role of chemotherapy

Currently, chemotherapy has no proven beneficial role in pontine gliomas. However, as the survival is so poor it is not surprising that there is great pressure, both from doctors and families of patients, to try to find effective agents. A phase 2 window model would seem attractive, with the activity of various combinations of drugs or, preferably, single agents being investigated before the use of radiotherapy. There are, however, real problems with a phase 2 window model. The use of chemotherapy before radiotherapy delays the only proven active treatment modality and can result in neurological deterioration that may not be relieved by steroids or radiotherapy. Also, phase 2 trials depend on showing a reduction in tumour size after the use of an active agent; this is often not possible in diffuse pontine gliomas as the differentiation of tumour from oedematous brain is difficult. Once patients relapse, many are in such poor condition or have such rapidly progressive disease that trials of new drug therapy are not appropriate. In the UK Childrens' Cancer Study Group we are starting a series of trials of new drug therapy with the agents being given along with radiotherapy. The agents will be those for which some evidence has been accrued in relapsed patients and the end-point is a shift in the median survival rather than tumour shrinkage.

Symptom care of patients with brain tumours

So far this chapter has concentrated on the controversies surrounding curative therapy in children with high-risk gliomas. However, irrespective of outcome in terms of cure, we have a responsibility to keep the discomfort of the disease to a minimum and, for the majority of patients who will die of their disease, to try to ensure a dignified and peaceful death. Most patients and their families now choose for the child to die at home rather than in hospital. Therefore, the families and local services have to be trained and supported in order for the children to receive optimal care. The availability of a local paediatric community nursing team, working with support from a specialist symptom-care team based at the oncology centre, is a huge help in achieving these aims. Symptom-care teams are made up of specialist nurses (with medical support) who visit patients in their homes and liaise with and advise local medical and nursing colleagues. Palliative care is an enormous topic and good reference books are available on the subject (Goldman, 1998). However, certain areas are contentious: the use of steroids, the management of various specific types of pain and the care of the child with increasing neurological handicap.

The role of steroids

It is vital to have an agreed policy for the use of steroids in children with brain tumours (Glaser *et al.*, 1997). The use of corticosteroids, usually dexamethasone, can be life saving in children with raised intracranial pressure and can preserve vital neurological function in children with spinal cord compression. Indeed, it would be negligent not to use steroids in these circumstances. The dosage in emergency situations is high, at 0.5–1.0 mg/kg daily in three divided doses. However, chronic administration leads to weight gain, hypertension, thinning of the skin, osteoporosis, mood changes, susceptibility to infection and adrenal suppression. One of the most tragic sights in neuro-oncology is the child with a brainstem glioma who is grossly cushingoid, sometimes to the extent that the child no longer recognises themselves in the mirror. The history in these circumstances is of neurological deterioration treated with an increase in steroids, followed by further neurological deterioration and further steroid dose increases. Eventually the child becomes moody, irritable or psychotic, with a raging hunger that they are unable to satisfy as their bulbar palsies progress to such an extent that they can no longer chew or swallow. In our unit, we use steroids for as short a period as possible, having discussed their use with parents early after diagnosis. In a child with progressive disease, a short course of steroids allows neurological stability so that a family visit or a favourite event can be enjoyed, but then the child is weaned off the steroids, even though the neurological state may deteriorate. For parents to wean a child off a drug while watching their child worsen is difficult and only achievable if it has been discussed in detail beforehand and the parents recognise that active measures will be taken to control pain and nausea.

Pain

In the brain tumour population, pain is either headache caused by raised intracranial pressure, nerve pain caused by direct invasion or pain from secondary phenomena such as muscle spasms, skin breakdown or constipation. As in the rest of oncology, successful management depends on making an accurate assessment of the cause, site and severity of the pain. The aim is to keep the patient pain free rather than treating pain once it has been allowed to develop. It is imperative to teach patients or their parents how to use various analgesics and give them supplies of the drugs to keep at home in order to prevent long delays in calling medical or nursing help. A stepwise escalation of drugs, starting with paracetamol, moving up to dihydrocodeine and then on to morphine is appropriate for many, though in a small minority of patients opioid analgesia will be required from the start. The starting doses of various preparations are shown in Table 8.2.

Headache

Oncology units pride themselves on being responsive to a child's pain and use strong analgesia early. However, if a child presents with acutely raised intracranial pressure, opioid analgesia should be used with extreme caution if at all. The hypoventilation opioids can produce leads to a rise in blood carbon dioxide levels, resulting in dilatation of the cerebral vasculature and a further increase in intracranial pressure. As the child slips into unconsciousness, staff may attribute this simply to sleepiness from the opioids and adequately controlled pain. The use of dexamethasone will lower the intracranial pressure

Table 8.2 Useful drugs in the symptom care of children with central nervous system tumours

Drug	Treatment regimen
Steroids	
Dexamethasone	0.5 mg/kg daily in three divided doses orally. Can be given intravenously as a 15 min infusion at 50% of the oral dose. These are starting doses and may need to be increased
Analgesics	
Paracetamol	For mild-to-moderate pain, given 4 to 6 hourly to a maximum of 4 doses a day; dosage varies with age Age <3 months 10–15 mg/kg Age 3 months to 1 year 60–125 mg Age 1–5 years 125–250 mg Age 6–12 years 250–500 mg
Codeine phosphate	3 to 6 mg/kg daily in four to six divided doses
Morphine sulphate	Starting doses: 1 mg/kg daily for younger than 1 year, 2 mg/kg daily for >1 year. This should be increased as necessary. Doses should be decreased if renal failure is present. If using slow-release preparations, always provide a short-acting opioid for breakthrough pain. Doses can be given orally or rectally. Give short-acting morphine up to six times a day and long-acting (MST) twice a day.
Diamorphine	If children are unable to tolerate oral or rectal morphine, a subcutaneous infusion of diamorphine can be used. It can be mixed with cyclizine to control nausea and vomiting (see below). Give as either 20 µg/kg/hr continuous infusion or as 33% of the total dose of oral morphine that had been given in previous 24 hours as an infusion to run over 24 hours (i.e. if the dose of oral morphine had been 36 mg over last 24 hours we would give 12 mg diamorphine as a subcutaneous infusion to run over 24 hours (0.5 mg/h)).

N.B. Remember to prescribe lactulose for children on opioid analgesia.

Table 8.2 *Continued*

Drug	Treatment regimen
Anti-emetics	
Ondansetron	Orally three times a day Age <1 year 1 mg Age 1–4 years 2 mg Age >4 years 4 mg Adult 8 mg
Cyclizine	Particularly good for emesis caused by raised intracranial pressure. Doses can be given orally or rectally. All oral and rectal doses can be given three times daily. The same total daily dose can be given by subcutaneous infusion and is compatible with diamorphine (can be mixed in the same syringe) Age <1 year 1 mg/kg/dose up to 3 times daily Age 1–4 years 12.5 mg/dose up to 3 times daily Age 4–12 years 25 mg/dose up to 3 times daily Age >12 years 50 mg/dose up to 3 times daily

and quickly reduce pain. In the setting of terminal care, however, the inverse applies, with the judicious use of opioids being far preferable to ever increasing steroid doses.

Nerve pain

Nerve pain is one of the most challenging symptoms to control as it often responds poorly to opioids. Therapy directed at controlling the underlying disease is often effective at relieving pain even in situations where the underlying condition cannot be cured; a few fractions of radiotherapy or the use of easily tolerated chemotherapy such as oral etoposide can be helpful. Drugs used primarily for the control of nerve pain include amitriptyline or carbamazepine, both in standard doses. Chronic pain 'sensitises' the nerves and in some patients even light touch on the affected area can produce excruciating discomfort. Agents such as ketamine can potentially reverse this sensitisation but should only be used on the advice of doctors specialising in pain control. For local or regional pain, an assessment by an anaesthetist specialising in pain control would be useful to determine whether there would be a role for nerve blocks or epidural analgesia. Many patients will try non-pharmacological measures such as transcutaneous electromagnetic nerve stimulation (TENS) or acupuncture, and some individuals appear to benefit though there are insufficient data to recommend that these therapies be used in standard practice.

Neurological dysfunction

Perhaps the most distressing part of neuro-oncology is the functional impairment of many of our patients. Children on therapy, or those whose disease is under control, should be given every opportunity to optimise their level of function, and teams of professionals including physiotherapists, occupational therapists, psychologists, speech therapists and orthopaedic surgeons are necessary. When a child has an incurable disease, the issues are different but a common mistake is not to offer any help, feeling it best 'to leave the child in peace'. Children love doing things and working hard to keep the child as functional as their disease state will allow is important. Simple measures such as teaching a child how to transfer from bed to wheel-chair, or from wheel-chair to toilet, will increase independence. In more severely affected children, concentrating on helping the child to feed themselves or to communicate is vital. Some children with brainstem gliomas can be almost 'locked in' as their tumour leads to quadriparesis and multiple cranial nerve palsies and yet intellectually they will remain aware and able to communicate.

Summary

Children with poor-risk glial tumours present a major challenge. It is imperative we develop more effective therapies in the context of properly conducted and published trials. However, not all patients and families will be willing to enter trials and many patients will be too ill to do so. Skilled symptom care is a prerequisite of any good neuro-oncology service.

Further reading

Boydston, W.R., Sanford, R.A., Muhlbauer, M.S. et al. (1991) Gliomas of the tectum and periaqueductal region of the mesencephalon. Pediatric Neurosurgery 17, 234–238.

Cairncross, G., Macdonald, D., Ludwin, S. et al. (1994) Chemotherapy for anaplastic oligodendroglioma. Journal of Clinical Oncology 12, 2013–2021.

Duffner, P.K., Horowitz, M.E., Krischer, J.P. et al. (1993) Postoperative chemotherapy and delayed radiation in children less than three years of age with malignant brain tumors. New England Journal of Medicine 328, 1725–1731.

Finlay, J.L., Boyett, J.M., Yates, A.J. et al. (1995) Randomised phase III trial in childhood high-grade astrocytoma comparing vincristine, lomustine and prednisone with the eight-drugs-in-1-day regimen. Journal of Clinical Oncology 13, 112–123.

Glaser, A.W., Buxton, N. and Walker, D. (1997) Corticosteroids in the management of central nervous system tumours. Archives of Disease in Childhood 76, 76–78.

Goldman, A. (ed.) (1998) Care of the Dying Child. Oxford: Oxford University Press.

Kadota, R.P. (1996) Perspectives on investigational chemotherapy and biologic therapy for childhood brain tumors. Journal of Pediatric Hematology/Oncology 18, 13–22.

Mason, W.P., Grovas, A., Halpern, S. et al. (1998) Intensive chemotherapy and bone marrow rescue for young children with newly diagnosed malignant brain tumors. Journal of Clinical Oncology 16, 210–221.

McCowage, G.B., Friedman, H.S., Moghrabi, A. et al. (1998) Activity of high-dose cyclophosphamide in the treatment of childhood malignant gliomas. Medical and Pediatric Oncology 30, 75–80.

Phuphanich. S., Edwards, M.S.B., Levin, V.A. et al. (1984) Supratentorial malignant gliomas of childhood. Results of treatment with radiation and chemotherapy. Journal of Neurosurgery 60, 495–499.

Rodriguez, R. and Kinsella, T.J. (1991) Halogenated pyrimidines as radiosensitisers for high grade glioma: revisited. International Journal of Radiation Oncology, Biology and Physics 21, 859–862.

Salazar, O.M., Rubin, P., Feldstein, M.L. et al. (1979) High dose radiation therapy in the treatment of malignant gliomas: final report. International Journal of Radiation Oncology, Biology and Physics 5, 1733–1740.

Sposto, R., Ertel, I.J., Jenkin, R.D.T. et al. (1989) The effectiveness of chemotherapy for treatment of high grade astrocytoma in children: results of a randomised trial. Journal of Neuro-oncology 7, 165–177.

CHAPTER 9

Germ cell tumours

E. Bouffet

Introduction

Primary CNS germ cell tumours (GCTs) are relatively rare and make up less than 3% of all brain tumours. Because of the rarity of CNS GCTs, published series usually combine both germinoma and non-germinomatous intracranial GCTs. Most of the information comes from retrospective analyses and very few prospective trials have been conducted. This may explain the amount of controversy in the management of these tumours. Discussion focusses around a number of issues, which are outlined below.

Management of germ cell tumours

Can we compare the data from cooperative groups? Comparisons between series are difficult. The main reason is that authors use two different methods to characterise patients with intracranial GCTs. Data are either based on the histological diagnosis from pathological specimens or on the secretion characteristics of the tumour. The histological diagnosis does not always match with tumour markers. This explains difficulties in comparing results when appropriate information is not available to translate from one system to another. When histological diagnosis is used, the term germinoma relates to tumours with an exclusive or predominant germinomatous component, regardless of the level of tumour markers. Tumours with different histology are usually grouped together as non-germinomatous GCTs but can also be defined as teratoma (regardless of the

tumour markers), mixed tumours or named according to the predominant histological component (embryonal carcinoma, yolk sac tumour, chorio-carcinoma, and mature or immature teratoma) or even called simply germinoma!

The problem is compounded by the possibility of low-level β human chorionic gonadotrophin (β-HCG) secretion in pure germinoma (without a chorio-carcinomatous component) containing occasional syncytiotrophoblastic cells (Shibamoto et al., 1997). The level of β-HCG used to define this subset of germinoma can vary according to the authors, despite a trend toward an accepted upper limit of 50 mIU/l. Moreover, patients with pure germinoma and negative tumour marker at diagnosis can present with elevated β-HCG at recurrence. Another difficulty concerns reports where the histological diagnosis is revised after second surgery following chemotherapy. The term teratoma is commonly used at that time, supporting the notion that chemotherapy has no influence on the mature teratomatous component when the tumour is heterogeneous.

When results are based on tumour secretion characteristics, germinomas are defined as histologically proven germinomas with negative tumour markers (allowing β-HCG level <50 mIU/l when germinomas with syncytiotrophoblastic cells are included). All other secreting tumours should be designated as secreting non-germinomatous GCTs. The use of standardised diagnostic nomenclature in future trials should be encouraged to avoid discrepancies in the eligibility criteria and to allow accurate comparisons of behaviour and outcome.

Is surgery required when tumour markers are positive?

Currently available imaging techniques will not provide accurate preoperative histological diagnosis of brain tumours, and surgical or stereotactical biopsy remains the standard approach to achieve a diagnosis. However, one-third of intracranial GCTs present with secretion of α-fetoprotein and/or HCG in the blood and the CSF. This may allow a diagnosis to be made without surgery. However, whether histological diagnosis is required when markers are initially positive remains controversial. Those favouring this approach point out that secreting tumours are morphologically heterogeneous, and the secretion often only accounts for a subset of the tumour tissue. Some authors even state that open biopsy (removing a large amount of tumour) is the procedure of choice, since small biopsy specimens could not include all of the components if the tumour is of mixed type (Ho and Liu, 1992). Another argument is that surgical debulking is a part of the standard treatment of most brain tumours, radical resection being associated with a better chance of survival. One argument against this is that surgical morbidity in suprasellar or pineal tumours is high, with a major risk of permanent neuroendocrine damage. Another argument against is that more accurate histological diagnosis does not influence the management of secreting tumours. Chemotherapy is the recognised treatment for intracranial secreting tumours, leading to dramatic tumour shrinkage in most cases. When chemotherapy is followed by focal or craniospinal irradiation, the 5-year survival is approximately 70% (Gobel et al., 1993; Baranzelli et al., 1997b). More accurate histological diagnosis would not change the type of chemotherapy used, and, therefore, there is little evidence that tissue diagnosis is mandatory for the management of secreting tumour.

Does the extent of surgery influence the outcome in CNS GCTs?

Classically, conservative management avoiding aggressive surgery was the policy for tumours of the pineal and suprasellar region. The recent development of microsurgical techniques has made major resection possible, and surgically orientated series have emphasised the role of extensive surgical removal.

There is, however, doubt that the extent of surgical resection influences outcome in patients with intracranial GCT. The complete plus subtotal resection rate in large series is generally low, precluding statistical evaluation of the impact of surgery on outcome: 18 out of 71 patients in the First International CNS Germ Cell Tumor Study Group trial (Balmaceda et al., 1996), 4 out of 18 in the SFOP protocol for NGGCT (Baranzelli et al., 1998a), 6 out of 57 in the SFOP study for germinomas (Bouffet et al., 1998) and 40% among 147 in the retrospective analysis from Matsumani et al. (1997). In this last series, seven patients died postoperatively, and nine additional patients exhibited major neurological complications.

Analysis of the influence of surgery on the outcome is difficult, since many retrospective series encompass periods with different means of assessment (operation notes, CT scan and MRI scan) and/or combine germinomas and non-germinomatous GCT in their analyses. Moreover, many groups disregarding surgery as a part of the initial management have used, and even still use, the 'radiation test' (Oi and Matsumoto, 1992) as a standard therapeutic regimen for tumours of the pineal and the suprasellar regions (i.e. if highly radiosensitive, conclude that it is a germinoma). Results of prospective trials do not favour an aggressive surgical approach. In the First International CNS Germ Cell Tumor Study Group trial (Balmaceda et al., 1996), patients with less than total resection showed a trend toward increased progression rate. However, this protocol did not include radiotherapy as a part of the initial management, and the progression rate was higher than expected. In the SFOP study for germinoma, the extent of surgery had no effect on progression-free and overall survival (Bouffet et al., 1998). Because of the poorer prognosis of secreting tumours, some authors recommend maximal resection to try and potentially improve local control. Recent data from cooperative groups suggest that a combined chemoradiotherapeutic approach produces a 60 to 70% overall survival rate (Gobel et al., 1993; Baranzelli et al., 1997b). Among variables likely to influence the outcome, no specific prognostic factor has yet been identified in prospective trials for secreting tumours.

In summary, there is no evidence that the extent of surgery influences the outcome in germinoma. The role of surgery in secreting tumours is poorly documented, but prospective trials do not suggest any impact on outcome. Despite technical advances, the morbidity of radical surgery is still high, leading to neurological or endocrine complications. Because of the efficacy of other treatments, surgical management should be as conservative as possible.

What is the role of chemotherapy?

The role of chemotherapy remains ill defined in intracranial GCTs. There is evidence that chemotherapy is effective both in germinoma and secreting tumours. However, the difference in curability between germinomas and secreting tumours has led to differing approaches in the management of these tumours.

Radiotherapy alone gives poor results in the treatment of secreting tumours. The introduction of neoadjuvant chemotherapy with regimens based on cyclophosphamide (or ifosfamide) and/or platinum compounds has led to a significant improvement in survival. The treatment results achieved in three consecutive German MAKEI protocols correlate with the cumulative dose of cisplatin (Calaminus *et al.*, 1994). In the MAKEI 89 protocol, patients received four cycles of ifosfamide–etoposide–cisplatin (cumulative dose: 400 mg/m^2) followed by craniospinal radiotherapy (Gobel *et al.*, 1993). The 4-year event-free survival rate in this trial was 75%. In the SFOP 1992 protocol, patients received six alternating courses of etoposide–carboplatin and etoposide–ifosfamide followed by focal irradiation (Bananzelli *et al.*, (1997b). The 4-year survival in this study was 76%. Although no randomised study has documented a survival advantage with chemotherapy, there is an overall agreement that chemotherapy has a major role in the management of secreting tumour.

By contrast, the respective role of chemotherapy and radiotherapy in germinoma remains a source of debate. Cure rates achieved with irradiation alone are high, and there is little evidence that combining chemotherapy and radiotherapy may lead to better survival. Groups favouring chemotherapy in germinoma primarily aim to reduce or to avoid radiotherapy. The experience of the First International CNS Germ Cell Tumor Study Group trial is questionable, since half of the germinoma patients required radiotherapy despite intensive chemotherapy that was associated with a significant toxic death rate (Balmaceda *et al.*, 1996). In the SFOP experience, chemotherapy was given for four courses and followed by a 40 Gy focal irradiation for patients with localised disease at diagnosis (Bouffet *et al.*, 1998). In 50 out of 51 patients with localised disease craniospinal prophylaxis was avoided. Three patients relapsed and achieved second remission using chemotherapy only (two patients) or chemotherapy followed by craniospinal irradiation (one patient). The overall survival in this group of patients is 100%. This experience suggests that chemotherapy might enable a reduction in the volume irradiated and, perhaps, also in the dose to the primary site.

Which drugs should be used?

Chemotherapy regimens have given rise to a number of questions. Should we use carboplatin or cisplatin? Should bleomycin be used? What is the role of ifosfamide?

Randomised trials conducted in adults with extracranial GCTs have shown that regimens using cisplatin at a dose of 100 mg/m^2 gave better progression-free rates than regimens with carboplatin at a dose of 400 or 500 mg/m^2. There are no data in the literature suggesting an advantage of either drug in intracranial GCTs. In intracranial germinoma and secreting non-germinomatous GCTs the response rate to cisplatin and carboplatin combinations is equivalent, in the range 80–100% (Table 9.1). The dose of carboplatin used in intracranial tumours is usually higher than cisplatin equivalent, in the range 600–1000 mg/m^2. Progression-free and overall survival do not seem to be influenced by the choice of the platinum compound but rather by the design of the protocols, including or avoiding adjunctive radiotherapy. The SFOP 88 protocol for non-germinomatous GCTs reported a high recurrence rate using carboplatin-based chemotherapy only (Baranzelli *et al.*, 1998a). The subsequent study incorporated focal irradiation and demonstrated a significant improvement, with a 76% overall survival (Baranzelli *et al.*, 1997b). The First International CNS Germ Cell Tumor Study Group trial achieved the same conclusions using a bleomycin–etoposide–carboplatin

Table 9.1 Response rates of intracranial germinoma and secreting non-germinomatous GCTs to cisplatin and carboplatin combinations

Author	Carboplatin	Cisplatin	Tumour type	Comments
Allen (1987)	1/2 G		G	
Baranzelli et al. (1997a)	15/18 responses		NGGCT	3 growing teratoma
Bouffet et al. (1998)	38/38 responses		G	
Balmaceda et al. (1996)	39/68 CR + 22/68 PR (89%)		G + NGGCT	4 PD (4 NGGCT) No radiotherapy
Plowman (1997)	6/7 G 4/5 NGGCT		G + NGGCT	
Allen (1994)	7/10 CR 3/10 PR		G	
Calaminus et al. (1997)		10/13 NGGCT	NGGCT	3 growing teratoma
Gobel et al. (1993)		16/21 OS	NGGCT	
Yoshida (1993)		G: 11/13 PR + CR NGGCT: 78% PR + CR	G + NGGCT	
Kobayashi (1989)		1/1 G 3/3 NGGCT	G + NGGCT	
Allen (1985)		4/7 G + NGGCT	G + NGGCT	
Castaneda (1990)		2/2 NGGCT	NGGCT	No radiotherapy
Chang (1995)		3/3 G 6/10 NGGCT	G + NGGCT	
Herrmann (1994)		3/3 NGGCT	NGGCT	
Robertson (1997)		5 CR 4 PR 2 SD 1 PD	NGGCT	
Sawamura (1998)		4/4 G 10/10 NGGCT	G + NGGCT	

G, germinoma; NGGCT, non-germinomatous germ cell tumour; CR, complete response; PR, partial response; PD, progressive disease; SD, stable disease; OS, overall survival.

regimen without irradiation, with a 50% relapse rate in both germinoma and non-germinoma patients (Balmaceda et al., 1996).

The role of bleomycin has also been emphasised in randomized trials including intermediate- and high-risk patients with extracranial GCTs. However, bleomycin's diffusion into brain is modest, and the role of this agent in intracranial GCTs is debatable. There are no data comparing regimens with and without bleomycin. Only one of the three reported prospective trials for patients with CNS GCTs (MAKEI, SFOP, First International CNS Germ Cell Tumor Study Group) used bleomycin (Gobel et al., 1993; Balmaceda et al., 1996; Baranzelli et al., 1998a; Bouffet et al.,

1998). The response rates in these trials are similar, but progression-free and overall survival show striking differences because of the radiotherapeutic design of these protocols. The toxic death rate in the First International CNS Germ Cell Tumor Study Group trial was significant (10%), but none of the patients developed recognised pulmonary toxicity.

Cyclophosphamide has shown an impressive activity in newly diagnosed or relapsed patients with intracranial GCT. It is, however, surprising to observe that no cooperative study has incorporated this agent in its first-line treatment. Ifosfamide has been incorporated in the MAKEI, the SFOP and the current SIOP protocol (Gobel et al., 1993; Baranzelli et al.,

1997b; Bouffet *et al.*, 1998; Calaminus *et al.*, 1994). Data on ifosfamide efficacy in intracranial GCT are few, although this drug has shown excellent CSF diffusion. The most important complication with ifosfamide in this clinical context is the destabilisation of diabetus insipidus in patients who are on hormone replacement (Bouffet *et al.*, 1998).

In summary, the choice of the platinum compound does not seem to influence the response rate in CNS GCTs. The role of bleomycin is unknown. The addition of ifosfamide rather than cyclophosphamide in the management of intracranial GCT is questionable.

Is craniospinal radiotherapy a standard treatment for germinomas?

Using craniospinal radiotherapy, the survival rate in large series of germinoma patients ranges between 75 and 95% (Matsumani *et al.*, 1997; Calaminus *et al.*, 1994). The usual prophylactic dose to the neuraxis in retrospective series ranges from 20 to 36 Gy, with a 40 to 60 Gy boost to the primary site. The toxicity of craniospinal radiotherapy is reported to be low, since the median age in germinoma patients is 11 to 12 years, and growth disturbances or intellectual side effects are less pronounced in older children. However, a significant proportion of patients with germinoma present with primary growth failure, and spinal irradiation may have an increased detrimental effect in children with growth impairment. Moreover, the rationale for this treatment is poor. The concept of craniospinal radiotherapy for germinoma was developed at a time when staging procedures were limited. With modern imaging procedures, accurate metastatic assessment is possible, and the proportion of patients presenting with metastatic disease at the time of diagnosis appears to be low. Furthermore, in a review of literature, Brada and co-workers (1990) have concluded that the incidence of secondary seeding did not differ between patients treated with craniospinal radiotherapy and those treated with whole brain radiotherapy. The benefit of systematic craniospinal radiotherapy, therefore, seems questionable. Recent studies have suggested that reduced doses of craniospinal radiotherapy are as effective (Shibamato *et al.*, 1994). Some authors favour reduced field and advocate irradiation to a generous local field encompassing the tumour site for localised germinomas. Others recommend that the radiotherapeutic management should include the ventricular radiation to 24–30 Gy with a boost to the primary tumour (Wolden *et al.*, 1995). The SFOP group has reported a 2-year overall survival of 100% in a group of 51 patients with localised germinoma treated with chemotherapy followed by focal irradiation at a dose of 40 Gy to the primary tumour bed, with a 1 cm safety margin (Bouffet *et al.*, 1998). Large variations are observed in the literature regarding the recommended dose to the primary site. Retrospective analyses have suggested a better outcome associated with doses above 40 Gy (Haddock *et al.*, 1997). New techniques such as radiosurgery or stereotactic radiotherapy are under investigation. It is plausible that reduced doses of radiotherapy similar to the doses used in seminomas in extracranial sites are sufficient to cure patients with the same histology. The current SIOP protocol is investigating two different approaches in a non-randomised trial. Arm A delivers low-dose craniospinal radiotherapy, and arm B four courses of etoposide–carboplatin-based chemotherapy followed by focal irradiation (40 Gy) to the primary site. No randomised study has yet been conducted to compare different radiotherapy modalities.

Is there a place for second-look surgery for residual disease after chemotherapy?

A significant proportion of patients present with residual radiographic abnormalities after initial treatment. With extracranial GCT, such residual radiographic abnormalities may be related to fibrous tissue, mature elements or viable tumour, and radiographic features cannot be used to exclude malignancy or teratoma reliably after chemotherapy. Based on this experience, some authors have suggested that patients with residual intracranial radiographic abnormalities should undergo surgical resection (Balmaceda *et al.*, 1996; Nashold *et al.*, 1994). In the First International CNS Germ Cell Tumor Study Group trial, nine patients underwent second-look surgery and six had no residual tumour (Balmaceda *et al.*, 1996). It is not stated whether the tumours were initially secreting or not. In the preliminary report of the SFOP experience with germinoma, nine patients had residual abnormality at treatment completion. No patients developed recurrence, with a median follow-up of 32 months (Baranzelli *et al.*, 1997a). The current SIOP trial for CNS GCTs recommends second-look surgery after chemotherapy and prior to irradiation for patients with secreting tumours who have residual abnormalities despite marker normalisation.

Second-look surgery may be considered when the primary tumour enlarges during chemotherapy, despite normalisation of tumour markers. The term 'growing teratoma syndrome' has been proposed to define this entity (O'Callaghan *et al.*, 1997). Histological examination of the resected tissue shows mature teratoma. It is suggested that the malignant elements of the tumour are responding to chemotherapy, while the mature teratoma component is not affected by chemotherapy and continues to grow, accounting for a paradoxical response to treatment. This complication accounts for three out of 13 patients in the cooperative German/Italian experience and three out of 18 patients in the SFOP one (Baranzelli *et al.*, 1998a; Calaminus *et al.*, 1997).

In summary, there is little information on the role of second-look surgery in CNS GCTs. One of the reasons might be the reluctance to operate on a small residue in the pineal or suprasellar area. Whether completeness of resection after chemotherapy may allow radiotherapy avoidance is still unproven.

What is the treatment for recurrent tumours?

The management for relapsing patients will vary according to the composition of the primary treatment. When the initial treatment did not include irradiation, radiotherapy is the treatment of choice. In a report describing eight patients with recurrent germinoma initially treated with carboplatin-based chemotherapy and no irradiation, Merchant and co-workers (1998) used high-dose cyclophosphamide followed by craniospinal radiotherapy. All patients achieved complete response and are free of disease, 16 to 47 following radiotherapy. In 1988, the SFOP group initiated a protocol based on chemotherapy only for patients with secreting tumours. Twelve of the thirteen non-irradiated patients relapsed. Treatment at the time of progression included chemotherapy in six patients and radiotherapy in 10. Six patients were salvaged, all but one with combined chemo- and radiotherapy (Baranzelli *et al.*, 1998a).

When initial treatment includes radiotherapy, re-irradiation may in some cases be possible. Ono and co-workers (1994) reported the treatment of nine patients who relapsed after radiotherapy; five developed disease in three non-irradiated sites. Four patients underwent surgery, four had further irradiation and three received chemotherapy. In this report, Ono divided recurrences into four groups, according to the site, the histology, and the pattern of secretion. Five patients survived, including two with benign recurrent teratoma and three who were re-irradiated.

The SFOP group has reported a pilot study of high-dose chemotherapy using etoposide and thiotepa for patients with recurrent CNS GCTs (Baranzelli *et al.*, 1998b). Thirteen patients were included, nine with an initial diagnosis of secreting tumour and four with germinoma. Ten patients responded to cisplatin-based salvage chemotherapy. At the time of high dose chemotherapy 6 patients were in complete remission, 4 were in partial remission and 3 had progressive disease. After a median follow-up of 16 months, all 10 responding patients were alive and in remission. Only three patients received additional radiotherapy. The three patients treated with evidence of progressive disease ultimately died. As in poor-risk or relapsed extracranial GCT, the role of high-dose chemotherapy remains to be defined.

Further reading

Allen, J.C., Kim, J.H. and Packer, R.J. (1987) Neoadjuvant chemotherapy for newly diagnosed germ-cell tumors of the central nervous system. *Journal of Neurosurgery* 67: 65–70.

Allen, J.C., Bosl, G. and Walker R. (1985) Chemotherapy trials in recurrent primary intracranial germ cell tumors. *Journal of Neurooncology* 3: 147–152.

Allen, J.C., Darosso, R., Donahue, B. and Nirenberg, A. (1994) A phase II trial of pre-irradiation carboplatin in newly diagnosed germinoma of the central nervous system. *Cancer* 74: 940–944.

Balmaceda, C., Heller, G., Rosenblum, M. *et al.* (1996) Chemotherapy without irradiation – a novel approach for newly diagnosed CNS germ cell tumors: results of an international cooperative trial. *Journal of Clinical Oncology* 14: 2908–2915.

Baranzelli, M.C., Patte, C., Bouffet, E. *et al.* (1997) Non-metastatic intracranial germinomas. The experience of the French Society of Pediatric Oncology. *Cancer* 80: 1792–1797.

Baranzelli, M.C., Patte, C., Thyss, A. *et al.* (1997b) Treatment of secreting intracranial germ cell tumour with carboplatin based chemotherapy and focal irradiation. *Medical and Pediatric Oncology* 29, 319 (abstract).

Baranzelli, M.C., Patte, C., Bouffet, E. *et al.* (1998a) An attempt to treat pediatric intracranial αFP and βHCG secreting germ cell tumors with chemotherapy alone. *Journal of Neuro-Oncology* 37: 229–239.

Baranzelli, M.C., Pichon, F., Patte, C. *et al.* (1998) High dose etoposide and thiotepa for recurrent intracranial malignant germ cell tumours. Experience of the French Society of Paediatric Oncology. Rome: 8th International Symposium on Pediatric Neuro-Oncology, May 6–9, 1998.

Bouffet, E., Baranzelli, M.C., Patte, C. *et al.* (1998) Combined treatment modality for intracranial germinomas. Results of a multicentre SFOP experience. *British Journal of Cancer*, in press.

Brada, M. and Rajan, B. (1990) Spinal seeding in cranial germinomas. *British Journal of Cancer* 61: 339–340.

Calaminus, G., Andreussi, L., Garre, M.L. *et al.* (1997) Sezernierende Keimzelltumoren des Zentralnerven-Systems (zns). Erste Ergebnisse der Kooperativen Deutsch/Italienischen Pilotstudie (CNS SGCT). *Klinische Pädiatrie* 209: 222–227.

Calaminus, G., Bamberg, M., Baranzelli, M.C. *et al.* (1994) Intracranial germ cell tumors: a comprehensive update of the European data. *Neuropediatrics* 25: 26–32.

Castaneda, V.L., Parmley, R.T., Geiser, C.F. *et al.* (1990) Postoperative chemotherapy for primary intracranial germ cell tumor. *Medical and Pediatric Oncology* 18: 299–303.

Chang, T.K., Wong, T.T. and Hwang, B. (1995) Combination chemotherapy with vinblastine, bleomycin, cisplatin, and etoposide (VBPE) in children with primary intracranial germ cell tumors. *Medical and Pediatric Oncology* 24: 368–372.

Gobel, U., Bamberg, M., Calaminus, G. *et al.* (1993) Verbesserte prognose intracranialer keimzelltumoren durch Intensivierte therapie: ergebnisse des therapieprotokolls MAKEI 89, *Klinische Pädiatrie* 205: 217–224.

Haddock, M.G., Schild, S.E., Scheithauer, B.W., Schomberg, P.J. (1997) Radiation therapy for histologically confirmed primary central nervous system germinoma. *International Journal of Radiation, Oncology, Biology and Physics* 38: 915–923.

Herrmann, H.D., Westphal, M., Winkler, K. *et al.* (1994) Treatment of non-germinomatous germ-cell tumors of the pineal region. *Neurosurgery* 34: 524–529.

Ho, D.M. and Liu, H.C. (1992) Primary intracranial germ cell tumor. Pathologic study of 51 patients. *Cancer* 70: 1577–1584.

Kobayashi, T., Yoshida, J., Ishiyama, J. *et al.* (1989) Combination chemotherapy with cisplatin and etoposide for malignant intracranial germ cell tumors. An experimental and clinical study. *Journal of Neurosurgery* 70: 676–681.

Matsumani, M., Sano, K., Takakura, K. *et al.* (1997) Primary intracranial germ cell tumors: a clinical analysis of 153 verified cases. *Journal of Neurosurgery* 86: 446–455.

Merchant, T.E., Davis, B.J., Sheldon, J.M. and Leibel, S.A. (1998) Radiation therapy for relapsed CNS germinoma after primary chemotherapy. *Journal of Clinical Oncology* 16: 204–209.

Nashold, J.R., Oakes, W.J., Friedman, H.S. *et al.* (1994) Management of pineal non-germinoma germ cell tumour with residual teratoma and normal alpha-fetoprotein. *Medical and Pediatric Oncology* 22: 137–139.

O'Callaghan, A.M., Katapodis, O., Ellison, D.W. *et al.* (1997) The growing teratoma syndrome in a non-germinomatous germ cell tumour of the pineal gland: a case report and review. *Cancer* 80: 942–947.

Oi, S. and Matsumoto, S. (1992) Controversies pertaining to therapeutic modalities for tumors of the pineal region: a worldwide survey of different patient populations. *Childs Nervous System* 8: 332–336.

Ono, N., Isobe, I., Uki, J. *et al.* (1994) Recurrence of primary intracranial germinomas after complete response with radiotherapy: recurrence patterns and therapy. *Neurosurgery* 35: 615–621.

Plowman, P.N., Kingston, J.E., Sebag Montefiore, D. and Doughty, D. (1997) Clinical efficacy of perceived 'CNS friendly' chemoradiotherapy for primary intracranial germ cell tumours. *Clin Oncol R Coll Radiol* 9: 48–53.

Robertson, P.L., DaRosso, R.C. and Allen, J.C. (1997) Improved prognosis of intracranial non-germinoma germ cell tumors with multimodality therapy. *Journal of Neurooncology* 32: 71–80.

Sawamura, Y., Shirato, H., Ikeda, J. *et al.* (1998) Induction chemotherapy followed by reduced-volume radiation therapy for newly diagnosed central nervous system germinoma. *Journal of Neurosurgery* 88: 66–72.

Shibamato, Y., Takahashi, M. and Abe, M. (1994) Reduction of the radiation dose for intracranial germinoma: a prospective study. *British Journal of Cancer* 70: 984–989.

Shibamoto, Y., Takahashi, M. and Sasai, K. (1997) Prognosis of intracranial germinoma with syncytiotrophoblastic giant cells treated by radiation therapy. *International Journal of Radiation Oncology, Biology and Physics* 37: 505–510.

Wolden, S.L., Wara, W.M., Larson, D.A. *et al.* (1995) Radiation therapy for primary intracranial germ-cell tumors. *International Journal of Radiation Oncology, Biology and Physics* 32: 943–949.

Yoshida, J., Sugita, K., Kobayashi, T. *et al.* (1993) Prognosis of intracranial germ cell tumours: effectiveness of chemotherapy with cisplatin and etoposide (CDDP and VP-16). *Acta Neurochir Wien* 120: 111–117.

CHAPTER 10
Ependymomas

E. Bouffet

Introduction

Ependymoma accounts for 6 to 12% of brain tumours in childhood. It represents the third most common brain tumour in this age range, following astrocytomas and medulloblastomas. Half of the cases occur in children before the age of 5 years, and most ependymomas arise in the posterior fossa. The management of this tumour remains controversial and may differ from surgery alone to a combination of surgery, chemotherapy and radiotherapy for the same tumour with the same histological diagnosis. The 5-year survival ranges between 30 and 50%, and most advances in the treatment of this tumour since the late 1970s have resulted from technical progress in surgical management. No real advance has been made using new strategies, such as intensive chemotherapy, or hyperfractionated radiotherapy. This chapter reviews some of the more contentious aspects of the management.

Management of ependymomas

Should the grading influence the treatment of ependymomas?

In general, increased malignancy is associated with a poorer outcome in oncology. There is, however, little evidence that the current grading system used for ependymomas has a prognostic value. Series in which anaplasia is associated with a poorer prognosis are either based on institutional classification or other non-WHO grading systems (Bouffet *et al.*, 1998). Series using the WHO grading system did not find an association between anaplasia and outcome. The most complex aspect of the histological grading in ependymoma is the huge variability in the percentage of anaplastic ependymomas between series. The average proportion of anaplastic ependymoma in the literature is 40 to 50%, ranging from 7 to 89% (Bouffet *et al.*, 1998)! This highlights the variation among pathologists in defining anaplastic ependymoma. The reasons why the current WHO classification fails to demonstrate a prognostic value in ependymoma are unclear. One reason may relate to the criteria that distinguish anaplastic ependymoma from ependymoma, particularly the proportion of anaplastic changes required to define anaplastic ependymomas. The association between histology and outcome may be confounded by age at diagnosis and the choice of therapy. One-third of childhood ependymoma occur before the age of two years, and infants are more likely to present with anaplastic tumours. Infants tend to fare worse than other children but the reasons cannot be restricted to the higher incidence of anaplastic variants. Tumours in infants are often larger than in older children and this may affect resectability (Figs. 10.1 and 10.2). Because of concerns regarding intellectual outcome, most of these infants are not irradiated or receive delayed irradiation. Although malignant histology may play a role in determining the poorer outcome of infants, resectability and the decision to defer or avoid potentially curative therapy may be an equally important factor.

Most of our knowledge regarding history and outcome is based on retrospective analyses, the

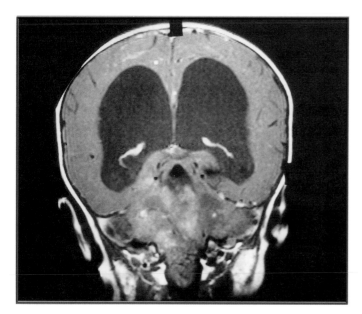

Figure 10.1 *Large posterior fossa ependymoma with massive hydrocephalus in a 1-year-old child.*

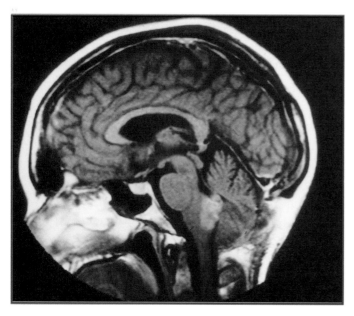

Figure 10.2 *Small posterior fossa ependymoma in a 16-year-old patient.*

pathology review often having been conducted by only one neuropathologist. Central pathology review in a recent report was associated with a 69% degree of discrepancy with the institutional diagnosis (Robertson *et al.*, 1998). Additional techniques may help to identify histological characteristics with a prognostic interest, such as Ki-67. Based on our current knowledge, there is little evidence that benign and anaplastic ependymoma should be treated differently.

What is the role of surgery in ependymomas?

Surgery has always been the mainstay of treatment for ependymoma and there is evidence that in some selected patients surgery alone can achieve cure. However, the influence of the extent of surgery on outcome has only been demonstrated recently in series where this has been accurately assessed by postoperative imaging. Series in which the extent of resection was based on operation notes or otherwise not clearly specified have often failed to highlight the role of surgery on outcome. In a study comparing imaging and clinical determination of the extent of surgery, the discrepancy rate was 32%, emphasising the difficulty of determining the extent of resection intraoperatively (Healey *et al.*, 1991). In the same study, the 10-year progression-free survival was 75% for patients having no radiological evidence of gross residual disease, compared with 0% for patients with postoperative residue on imaging. Several authors have confirmed this striking difference in either event-free or overall survival according to the extent of surgery. Since the mid-1980s, the importance of surgery in ependymoma has influenced the management of this disease, leading to the concept of aggressive surgery or, more recently, second-look surgery. Aggressive surgery carries with it a risk of significant morbidity, for example the need for temporary tracheostomy or prolonged enteral feeding in children with lateral ependymoma of the posterior fossa extending toward the cranial nerves. There is no evidence that this aggressive approach in extensive tumours improves survival, and postoperative morbidity might conversely delay postoperative treatment and reduce the chance of cure. Second-look surgery, possibly following chemotherapy, is at an early stage, and little information is available. It seems that this approach might reduce the morbidity and increase the complete resection rate, but its benefit for survival has still to be demonstrated (Foreman *et al.*, 1997).

Do we have to consider systematic radiotherapy, even after complete resection?

Postoperative radiotherapy is a part of the standard management of intracranial ependymomas. However, the evidence that radiotherapy benefits patients with ependymoma is slim. Regardless of their postoperative management, the outcome is uniformly poor for patients following incomplete resection (Healey *et al.*, 1991; Pollack *et al.*, 1995). There are no randomised data suggesting a survival advantage for postoperative radiotherapy. Series that support the use of postoperative radiotherapy do not analyse the reasons why patients were or were not irradiated. This may induce a bias, since poor postoperative recovery, advanced tumour, or young age may influence postoperative management. Nevertheless, there is a consensus to consider postoperative radiotherapy for children above 3 years of age. The experience of 'baby brain' protocols may help to clarify the role of radiotherapy. In these protocols, infants receive postoperative chemotherapy followed or not by delayed radiotherapy. Results of this approach are still preliminary, but the incidence of relapses in non-irradiated patients, even after complete resection, argues for a benefit of radiotherapy.

By contrast, reports on long-term survival following radical surgical treatment support a place for deferring adjuvant treatment. In a retrospective study of 12 paediatric patients with completely resected low-grade supratentorial ependymoma treated over a 30-year period, Palma and colleagues (1993) described four long-term survivors treated with surgery alone. Awaad and co-workers (1996) described seven patients with completely resected low-grade tumour who participated in a study of deferral of adjuvant therapy. Five patients remained free of progression 24 to 70 months following surgery. The term low grade was based on an institutional classification in both series. These reports concern highly selected patients, accounting for a small proportion of ependymoma patients. Criteria for selecting patients eligible for deferral of radiotherapy are missing. The literature experience suggests that a subset of patients with small hemispheric 'low-grade' tumours can avoid radiotherapy after complete resection. For tumours located in other sites, this approach remains experimental.

Does the technique and the extent of radiotherapy influence the outcome?

The most controversial question related to radiotherapy for ependymoma is the appropriate treatment volume. Until recently, treatment volume recommendations have been based on a perceived risk of seeding in this tumour, and craniospinal radiotherapy has been advocated for all types of ependymoma, or at least for the anaplastic variant. The incidence of primary or secondary seeding is, however, poorly documented and no series has prospectively assessed neuraxis dissemination at the time of relapse. Retrospective series have indicated that prophylactic spinal irradiation does not influence the incidence of spinal seeding, even in anaplastic tumours (Vanuytsel and Brada, 1991; Goldwein *et al.*, 1991).

The primary mode of failure in ependymoma remains disease recurrence at the primary site. Neuraxis dissemination when present is generally associated with local recurrence, and isolated spinal seeding or intracranial metastases are exceptional (Fig. 10.3a,b). Based on current knowledge, the treatment volume for radiotherapy should be the primary tumour bed with safety margins. However, several groups still consider craniospinal radiotherapy as the standard treatment, at least for so-called malignant ependymomas.

A dose–response relationship has been suggested from retrospective analyses, with a better local control for patients receiving more than 45 Gy to the primary site. In these series, the reasons to use different radiation parameters in a cohort of patients with the same histology have not been assessed, and no firm conclusions can be drawn from the present literature regarding the appropriate dose of radiotherapy in ependymoma. However, the importance of tumour control has led to innovative approaches in treatment delivery, such as hyperfractionation, stereotactic radiotherapy, or radiosurgery boost following conventional radiotherapy. Results of these experiences are pending.

Is there a place for chemotherapy in the standard management?

Information regarding the role of chemotherapy in ependymoma is poor. There is only one randomised trial comparing postoperative radiotherapy to radiotherapy followed by chemotherapy and this failed to demonstrate a survival advantage for chemotherapy (Evans *et al.*, 1996). Phase II data come from broad phase II studies that generally have included a small number of ependymoma patients. The overall response rate to single agents is in the range 15–20%,

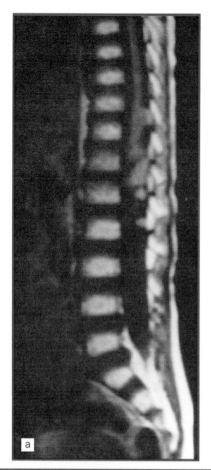

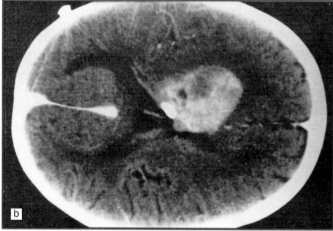

Figure 10.3 *Spinal (a) and supratentorial (b) seeding of a low-grade ependymoma of the posterior fossa.*

(Duffner *et al.*, 1993). Combinations that have demonstrated promising activity in medulloblastoma, such as MOPP, the '8 in 1' or the etoposide–carboplatin regimen give disappointing results in ependymomas. The experience of high-dose chemotherapy, although limited, does not support a dose–effect relationship in this tumour. All but one series in which the role of chemotherapy has been retrospectively assessed failed to demonstrate a benefit of chemotherapy. The only report suggesting a survival advantage with chemotherapy does not provide any response rate to document its efficacy (Needle *et al.*, 1997). Apart from the POG experience, use of 'baby-brain protocols' is not supporting the role of chemotherapy in infants with incompletely resected tumours. The role of chemotherapy in ependymoma remains highly critical. Because of the disappointing results obtained in this tumour, the decision-making process has introduced chemotherapy into the standard management of most children with intracranial ependymoma. As the benefit of adjuvant chemotherapy (either with or without radiotherapy) to individual patients is difficult to determine, prospective randomised trials are necessary to document improvements in relapse-free and overall survival.

What is the best treatment at the time of progression?

Ependymoma is a surgically-controlled disease. Surgery is still the best option at the time of progression (Goldwein *et al.*, 1990). Since local recurrence is the primary manifestation of treatment failure, reoperation should be considered when the surgeon feels that complete clearance can be achieved with little morbidity. When complete resection is possible, the role of adjuvant chemotherapy is questionable (see above). For children with incomplete resection or unresectable tumours, the use of chemotherapy can be considered with the aim of reducing the tumour volume and allowing further surgery. The experience of re-irradiation is still limited, but promising results have been reported with radiosurgery, particularly for small recurrences.

The role of surgery at the time of progression and the possibility of successful re-irradiation for small recurrences emphasises the importance of the early

with very few complete responses. Data from the literature suggest that cisplatin is the most effective single agent, with a 30% response rate. Surprisingly, other platinum compounds such as carboplatin or iproplatin are not effective. Combinations do not give better response rates, apart from the vincristine and cyclophosphamide regimen from the baby POG experience, with an amazing 48% response rate

detection of relapses in ependymoma. The correlation between early detection and improved outcome remains unclear in the majority of brain tumours. Ependymomas may differ from other malignant brain tumours because of the possibility of achieving complete surgical clearance when relapse occurs at the primary site.

Is there a specific management for ependymomas in infants?

Concerns regarding the cognitive and neuroendocrine consequences of radiotherapy in young children have led to the concept of baby-brain protocols, aiming to defer or avoid radiotherapy. Institutional or co-operative protocols are currently used worldwide, with a flexible upper limit for eligibility ranging from 3 to 6 years of age. These protocols differ in their design but share the same characteristics: they are based on a 4 to 6 drug regimen given after the initial operation over a 1 to 3 year period. The experience of these protocols in ependymoma is still poorly documented. The POG initiated in 1985 a protocol using a four-drug regimen until the age of 3 years, followed by craniospinal radiotherapy for medulloblastoma and ependymoma patients (Duffner *et al.*, 1993). The 5-year survival for infants with ependymomas is 40%. Prognostic factors in this experience are the extent of surgery and the age, with a poorer outcome for children less than 1 year, regardless of the extent of surgery. This suggests that delayed radiotherapy may affect the outcome. The follow-up period of other co-operative protocols (such as UKCCSG or SFOP) is too short to draw clear conclusions. It is noticeable that the POG, which has the longest experience in this area, is currently reconsidering the age limit to give radiotherapy. Children aged 18 months and above are currently eligible for pilot studies using conformal or stereotactic radiotherapy.

Further reading

Awaad, Y.M., Allen, J.C., Miller, D.C. *et al.* (1996) Deferring adjuvant therapy for totally resected intracranial ependymoma. *Pediatric Neurology* 14: 216–219.

Bouffet, E., Perilongo, G., Canete, A. and Massimino, M. (1998) Intracranial ependymomas in children. A critical review of the prognostic factors and a plea for cooperation. *Medical and Pediatric Oncology* 30: 319–331.

Duffner, P.K., Horowitz, M.E., Krischer, J.P. *et al.* (1993) Postoperative chemotherapy and delayed radiation in children less than three years of age with malignant brain tumors. *New England Journal of Medicine* 328: 1725–1731.

Evans, A.E., Anderson, J.R., Lefkowitz Boudreaux, I.B. and Finlay, J.L. (1996) Adjuvant chemotherapy of childhood posterior fossa ependymoma: cranio-spinal irradiation with or without adjuvant CCNU, vincristine, and prednisone: A Childrens Cancer Group study. *Medical and Pediatric Oncology* 27: 8–14.

Foreman, N.K., Love, S., Gill, S. and Coakham, H. (1997) Second look surgery for incompletely resected fourth ventricle ependymomas: technical case report. *Neurosurgery* 40: 856–860.

Goldwein, J.W., Glauser, T.A., Packer, R.J. *et al.* (1990) Recurrent intracranial ependymomas in children: survival, patterns of failure, and prognostic factors. *Cancer* 66: 557–563.

Goldwein, J.W., Corn, B.W., Finlay, J.L. *et al.* (1991) Is craniospinal irradiation required to cure children with malignant (anaplastic) intracranial ependymomas? *Cancer* 67: 2766–2771.

Healey, E.A., Barnes, P.D., Kupsky, W.J. *et al.* (1991) The prognostic significance of postoperative residual tumor in ependymoma. *Neurosurgery* 28: 666–672.

Needle, M.N., Goldwein, J.W., Grass, J. *et al.* (1997) Adjuvant chemotherapy for the treatment of intracranial ependymoma of childhood. *Cancer* 80: 341–347.

Palma, L., Celli, P., Cantori, G. *et al.* (1993) Supratentorial ependymomas of the first two decades of life. Long-term follow-up of 20 cases (including two subependymomas). *Neurosurgery* 32: 169–175.

Pollack, I.F., Gerszten, P.C., Martinez, A.J. *et al.* (1995) Intracranial ependymomas of childhood: Long-term outcome and prognostic factors. *Neurosurgery* 37: 665–667.

Robertson, P.L., Zeltzer, P.M., Boyett, J.M. *et al.* (1998) Survival and prognostic factors following radiation therapy and chemotherapy for ependymomas in children: a report of the Children's Cancer Group. *Journal of Neurosurgery* 88: 695–703.

Vanuytsel, L.J. and Brada, M. (1991) The role of prophylactic spinal irradiation in localized intracranial ependymoma. *International Journal of Radiation Oncology, Biology and Physics* 21: 825–830.

PART III
Solid tumours

CHAPTER 11

Neuroblastoma

C.R. Pinkerton

Introduction

Neuroblastoma has been the subject of considerable study with regard to molecular pathogenesis and is one of the first childhood cancers in which molecular pathology has been incorporated in treatment decisions. It is becoming clear that in the past many children have received unnecessarily intensive treatment and much effort has gone into improving prognostic stratification in localised disease. Conversely, the treatment of advanced disease remains frustrating, with high relapse rates despite initial chemosensitivity.

Diagnostic criteria

In an attempt to standardise definitions, the INSS produced sets of clinical criteria. These are shown in Box 11.1. The imaging modality used to document the primary site depends to some extent on the need, or otherwise, for precise tumour dimension measurement. Where the child is treated on an investigational protocol, two- or three-dimensional measurement may be a prerequisite, in which case detailed high-resolution imaging may be required (Fig. 11.1). If not, ultrasound is perfectly adequate to document the site and approximate dimensions. The main limitation with ultrasound is the difficulty in central review of the image and interpretation of the ultrasound information from photographic copies. The introduction of MRI has largely obviated the need for CT myelography. In the past, this procedure was

---

Box 11.1 Diagnosis of neuroblastoma

Neuroblastoma is diagnosed if one of the two following conditions is fulfilled:

1. Unequivocal pathologic diagnosis[a] is made from tumour tissue by light microscopy (with or without immunohistology, electron microscopy, increased urine or serum catecholamines or metabolites[b])

2. Bone marrow aspirate or trephine biopsy contains unequivocal tumour cells[a] (e.g. syncytia or immunocytologically positive clumps of cells) and increased urine or serum catecholamines or metabolites[b])

---

[a] If histology is equivocal, karyotypic abnormalities in tumour cells characteristic of other tumours [e.g. t(11;22)] then exclude a diagnosis of neuroblastoma, whereas genetic features characteristic of neuroblastoma (1p deletion, N-*myc* amplification) would support this diagnosis.

[b] Catecholamines and metabolites include dopamine, HVA and/or VMA; levels must be >3.0 SD above the mean per milligram creatinine for age to be considered increased, and at least two of these must be measured.

---

used with paraspinal tumours to document any intraspinal extension. Although this may have been apparent on high-resolution CT scan, without intrathecal contrast this was not always the case (Figs. 11.2 and 11.3).

The skeletal survey has now been replaced by the use of technetium isotope scan. There is rarely any doubt about the nature of bone scan abnormalities in metastatic neuroblastoma, but where the number of metastases are limited, plain X-ray of the involved bone may be of diagnostic help. Increasingly, mIBG scanning has come to replace technetium and has the advantage of tumour specificity (Figs. 11.4 and 11.5).

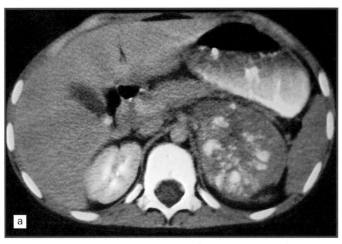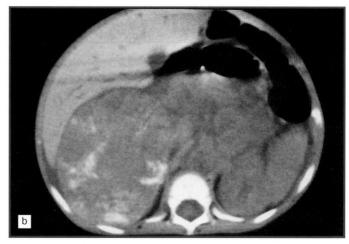

Figure 11.1 *CT scans showing calcified suprarenal masses. (a) Relatively localised tumour with little infiltration around the great vessels. (b) Extensive local spread and node involvement.*

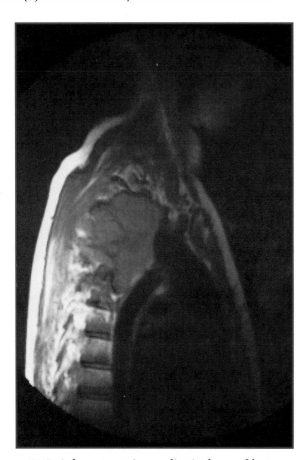

Figure 11.2 *A large posterior mediastinal neuroblastoma with infiltration into the vertebral column.*

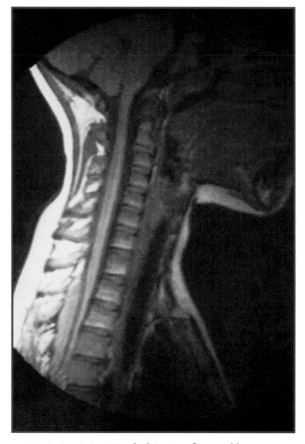

Figure 11.3 *An intraspinal deposit of neuroblastoma causing upper cord compression.*

There is continued debate regarding the distinction between mIBG uptake in the bone marrow cavity and the cortical bone. This may seem of only academic importance, but in view of the fact that bone positivity, as opposed to bone marrow positivity, may be an independent adverse prognostic factor, this distinction may be important.

Methods used to evaluate bone marrow have also been an area of contention. It is now agreed that a single aspirate may be adequate to confirm the diagnosis in a child with heavily involved marrow but is entirely inadequate to exclude marrow disease or assess response. Multiple single aspirates (up to 10) with examination of pooled buffy coat preparations

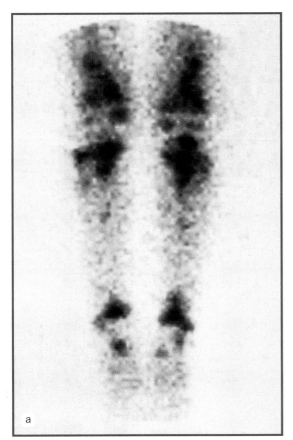

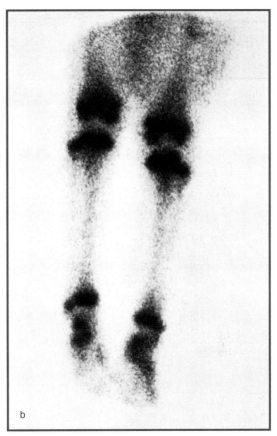

Figure 11.4 *mIBI scanning (a) and technetium scan (b) in lower limb of Stage 4 neuroblastoma.*

are comparable to bilateral aspirates and trephines (Fig. 11.6). Studies have evaluated the relevance of quantitative cytology, and the extent of marrow involvement appears to be an independent adverse prognostic factor. Such detailed analysis is not, however, required for standard practice.

Pathology

Several classifications have been developed, all claiming to be of prognostic value. The most widely used is the Joshi classification (Table 11.1) and, more recently, the Shimada classification (Table 11.2; Figs.

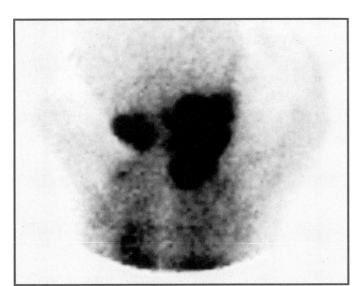

Figure 11.5 *mIBI uptake in an unusual extensive localised cervical ganglioneuroblastoma.*

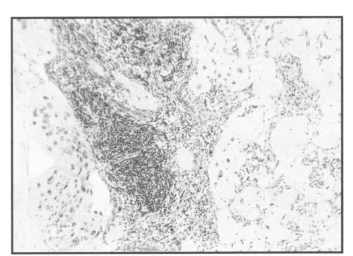

Figure 11.6 *Bone marrow infiltration on trephine.*

Table 11.1 Pathological subtypes of neuroblastic tumours: the Joshi classification

Tumour type	Characteristics	Subgroups
Neuroblastoma	>50% neuroblasts	Undifferentiated
		Poorly differentiated
		Differentiating
Ganglioneuro-blastoma	>50% ganglioneuro-matous	Nodular
		Intermixed
		Borderline
Ganglioneuroma	Mature ganglion cells	
	Neurites and	
	Schwann cell	
	No mitoses	

Table 11.2 Neuroblastic tumour subtypes: the Shimada classification system

Type of neuroblastic tumour	Favourable histology	Unfavourable histology
Neuroblastoma, stroma-rich(SR): age <5 years	Well-differentiated subtype: intermixed subtype	Nodular subtype (all ages)
Neuroblastoma, stroma-poor (SP)		
age ≤1.5 years	MKI<200	MKI >200
age 1.5–5 years	MKI <100 and differentiating	MKI >100 or undifferentiated
age >5 years	None	All

MKI, mitosis–karyorrhexis index.

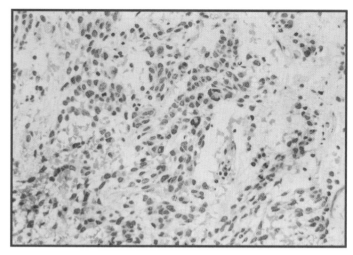

Figure 11.7 *Undifferentiated neuroblastoma.*

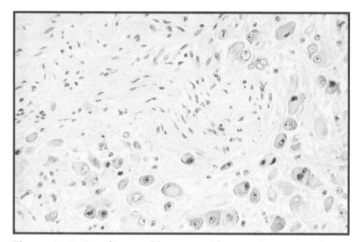

Figure 11.8 *Ganglioneuroblastoma with extensive neuronal differentiation.*

11.7 and 11.8). The Neuroblastoma Study Group has formed to provide a consensus. The Shimada classification has been somewhat contentious because of the difficulty in standardisation and because of its complexity. It has the advantage of taking into account clinical factors such as age, but with the application of biological prognostic factors has not gained popularity. Other groupings have attempted to combine clinical and biological characteristics (Table 11.3).

Immunophenotyping is a prerequisite and can be done on bone marrow aspirate, and on fixed or frozen tissue. The antibodies commonly used include non-specific esterase (NSE) and P-gp 1.5 (Fig. 11.9). In difficult cases there may be a role for electron microscopy, although as this technique may not be readily available it is not currently widely used. Demonstration of neurosecretory granules may confirm the origin of the tumour (Fig. 11.10).

Molecular pathology

The features that have now been clearly demonstrated to influence prognosis are listed in Table 11.3. Unfortunately, it has taken several years for sufficiently large prospective studies to be performed using standard methodology and treatment in order to document the unequivocal independent prognostic impact of N-*myc* amplification. Methods used to document N-*myc* include:

Table 11.3 Grouping of clinical and genetic types of neuroblastoma as related to prognosis (Brodeur)

Features	Type 1	Type 2	Type 3
Karyotype and ploidy	Hyperdiploid near triploid	Diploid/tetraploid	Tetraploid
Chromosome 1p	Normal	Normal	Deleted
N-*myc*	Normal	Normal	Amplified
LDH	Normal	<5 times elevated	Increased
Ferritin	Normal	<150 mg/ml	>150 mg/ml
Age	<12 months	Any	Any age
Stage	1, 2, 4S	3, 4	Any stage
Shimada	Good	Any	Bad
Outcome	Good	Intermediate	Bad

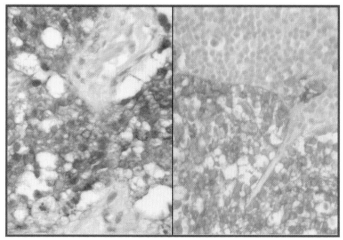

Figure 11.9 *Standard immunological marker positivity on biopsy. (NSE, PGP 1.5).*

- Southern analysis: this is the gold standard technique but requires substantial quantities of DNA, which may not be readily available for diagnostic samples.
- RT–PCR: this requires minimal tissue but is subject to laborotory variation and there may be problems with quantification.
- Fluorescence in-situ hybridisation (FISH): in experienced hands N-*myc*-specific probes produce the clearest and most unequivocal evidence of N-*myc* amplification, require limited numbers of cells and have increasingly become the method of choice (Figs. 11.11–11.13).

Detection of N-*myc* protein using either Western analysis or immunohistochemistry has been limited by the availability of suitable antibodies.

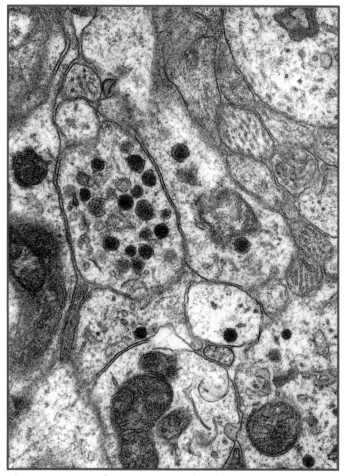

Figure 11.10 *Electronmicrograph showing neurosecretory granules.*

As with most solid tumours, a standard karyotype is difficult to establish and, therefore, FISH has revolutionised the ability to document deletion of part of chromosome 1. It also has the advantage of facilitating documentation of N-*myc* amplification

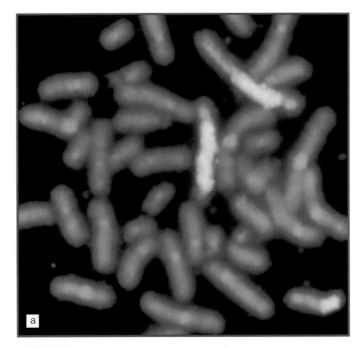

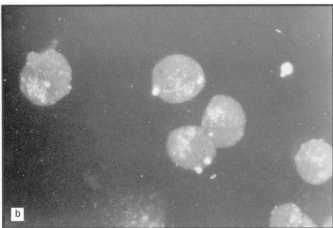

Figure 11.11 *N*-myc *amplification using fluorescent* in situ *hybridisation (FISH). (a) In metaphase spread; (b) an interphase preparation.*

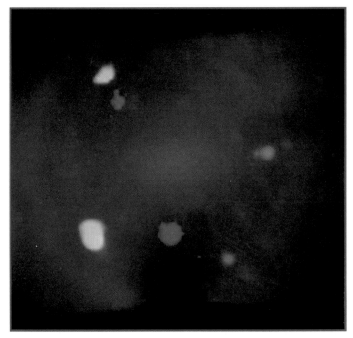

Figure 11.12 *Neuroblastoma without adverse molecular prognostic factors. No evidence of N-myc amplification (red). Two normal copies of chromosome 1p36 in blue and 1q11 in green.*

simultaneously in a single specimen. Deletions on chromosome 17 now also appear to be of adverse prognostic significance.

Diploid and tetraploid tumours appear to do worse, but standardisation of methodology has limited the use of this feature. Similarly, detection of P-gp or MDR1 gene overexpression may be associated with high-risk neuroblastoma. The methods of detection – immunohistochemistry, Northern analysis and quantitative RT–PCR – vary widely and most studies involve small numbers of patients. More recently, high levels of multidrug resistance protein (MRP) have been shown to correlate with a poor prognosis.

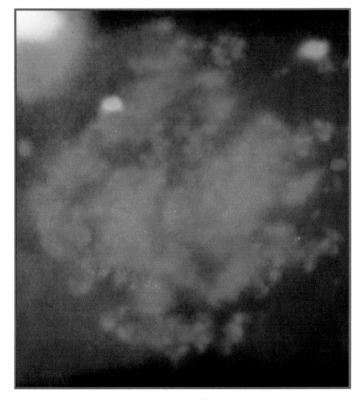

Figure 11.13 *Biology indicative of high-risk neuroblastoma with extensive N-myc amplification in red. Normal chromosome 1p36 (in blue).*

Staging

Often the presence of distant metastases is clear (Figs. 11.14 and 11.15). Three staging systems have been used: the St Jude classification, POG classification and the ENSG. The INSS have now produced a standardised classification that can be utilised by all groups (Table 11.4). This is a prerequisite to enabling useful comparison of clinical studies, which has been difficult because of variations in terminology. Figure 11.16 shows Stage 2 ganglioneuroblastomas. With the advances made with regard to tumour biology and diagnostic imaging, this classification has required regular updating and there remain a number of contentious issues. Definition of midline should be noted. It is now acceptable to have intraspinal extension to the lateral spinal border but remain Stage 2. Scanning of bone and bone marrow with mIBG is now included and an attempt has been made to quantify the extent of bone marrow involvement in Stage 4S disease using mIBG. The latter is probably inappropriate, as, if anything, mIBG is more sensitive than standard histology or cytology and will, therefore, detect minimal, not extensive, marrow infiltration. At present, none of the biological factors mentioned

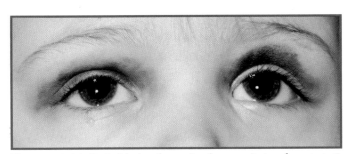

Figure 11.14 *Periorbital echymosis characteristic of metastatic neuroblastoma.*

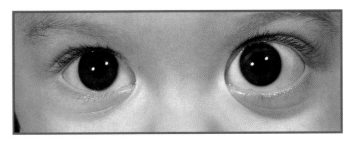

Figure 11.15 *Right-sided ptosis and exophthalmos caused by retro-orbital infiltration in metastatic neuroblastoma.*

Table 11.4 International staging system for neuroblastoma (INSS)

Stage	Characteristics
1	Localised tumour with complete gross excision, with or without microscopic residual disease; representative ipsilateral and contralateral lymph nodes negative for tumour microscopically (nodes attached to and removed with the primary tumour may be positive)
2a	Localised tumour with incomplete gross excision; representative ipsilateral and non-adherent lymph nodes negative for tumour microscopically
2b	Localised tumour with complete or incomplete gross excision; with ipsilateral non-adherent lymph nodes positive for tumour; enlarged contralateral lymph nodes must be negative microscopically
3	Unresectable unilateral tumour infiltrating across the midline with or without regional lymph node involvement; or localised unilateral tumour with contralateral regional lymph node involvement; or midline tumour with bilateral extension by infiltration (unresectable) or by lymph node involvement
4	Any primary tumour with dissemination to distant lymph nodes, bone, bone marrow, liver, skin and/or other organs (except as defined in Stage 4S)
4S	Localised primary tumour (as defined for Stage 1, 2a or 2b) with dissemination limited to skin, liver and/or bone marrow (limited to infants less than 1 year old)

above are routinely incorporated in staging, but it seems likely that in the near future a new classification will be developed.

Treatment strategies

There is little difference in outcome with localised tumours that are completely resected or those with microscopic residue. Adjuvant chemotherapy or local radiotherapy are not required. At the present time, there is insufficient evidence to warrant treatment intensification in these cases on the basis of biological features, but ultimately this may change. Table 11.5 lists the response-to-treatment criteria developed by the INSS and Figure 11.17 is an algorithm for the

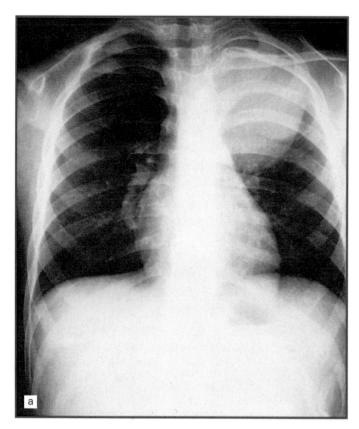

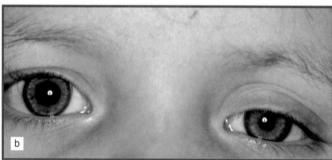

Figure 11.16 *Posterior mediastinal mass caused by Stage 2 ganglioneuroblastoma. (a) Well-circumscribed posterior mass, typical of low-risk disease; (b) left-side Horner's syndrome.*

Table 11.5 INSS response to treatment criteria

Response	Primary tumour[a]	Metastatic sites[a,b]
CR	No tumour	No tumour; catecholamines normal
VGPR	Decreased by 90–99%	No tumour; catecholamines normal; residual ^{99}Tc-detected bone changes allowed
PR	Decreased by >50%	All measurable sites decreased by >50%; bones and bone marrow: number of positive bone sites decreased by >50%; no more than one positive bone marrow site allowed[b]
MR	No new lesions; >50% reduction of any measurable lesion (primary or metastases) with <50% reduction in any other; <25% increase in any existing lesion	
NR	No new lesions; <50% reduction but >25% increase in any existing lesion	
PD	Any new lesion; increase of any measurable lesion by >25%; previous negative marrow positive for tumour	

[a] Evaluation of primary and metastatic disease.

[b] One positive marrow aspirate or biopsy allowed for PR if this represents a decrease from the number of positive sites at diagnosis.

CR, complete response; VGPR, very good partial response; PR, partial response; MR, minimal response; NR, no response; PD, progressive disease.

management of Stage 2 tumours with intraspinal extension. Decision regarding whether laminectomy or radiotherapy is used is to a large extent age dependent and may be influenced by the duration or extent of neurological deficit (Fig. 11.2). Whether laminectomy reduces late sequelae remains to be shown (Fig. 11.18).

Primary intracranial tumours are an unusual site (Fig. 11.19). Surgical excision, if possible, is treatment of choice, followed by local radiotherapy. A decision regarding radiotherapy and chemotherapy will depend on the degree of differentiation and biology of the tumour.

Management of Stage 3 tumours has been most markedly influenced by advances in tumour biology. It is now clear that those with N-*myc* amplification behave like Stage 4 tumours and require more intensive treatment. Conversely, those without adverse biological features may more closely resemble Stage 2 tumours and require little, if any, treatment. There is a recent trend towards managing these patients in the same way as Stage 2, i.e. surgical excision where feasible without any subsequent chemotherapy or radiotherapy. In some situations large tumours have been simply observed and have not progressed (Fig. 11.20).

The management of N-*myc*-positive patients is outlined in Figure 11.21. The intensity of chemo-

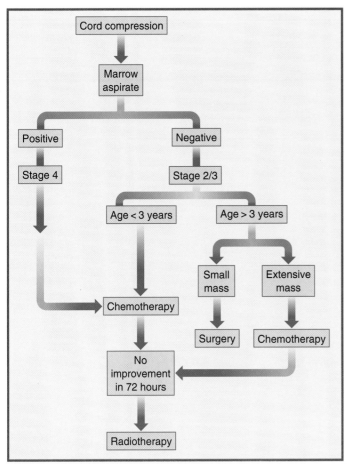

Figure 11.17 *Algorithm for the management of acute cord compression in neuroblastoma.*

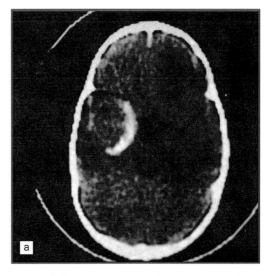

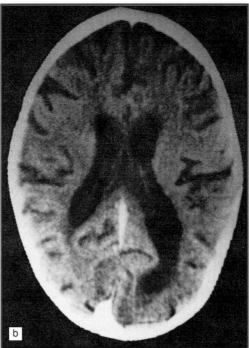

Figure 11.19 *(a, b) Examples of primary intracerebral neuroblastoma.*

therapy varies between national protocols, but it seems logical to apply regimens comparable to those used for Stage 4 patients.

The issue of what to do with incompletely resected tumour after chemotherapy continues to pose problems. Treatment options are outlined in Figure 11.22.

Stage 4 disease

Outcome in Stage 4 disease remains disappointing, with less than one-fifth of patients alive at 5 years. Despite many attempts to intensify treatment or introduce alternative chemotherapy agents, little

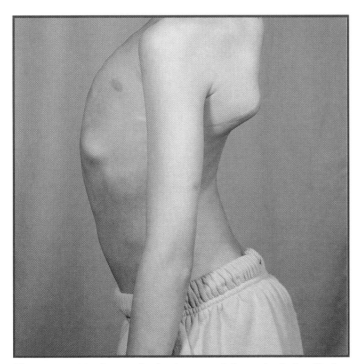

Figure 11.18 *Severe kyphosis caused by spinal irradiation combined with two laminectomies. Associated with repeated therapy of local recurrent ganglioneuroblastoma.*

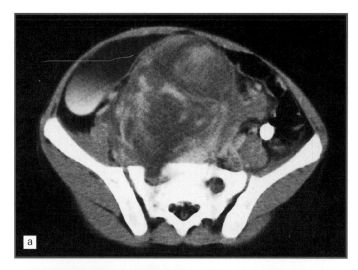

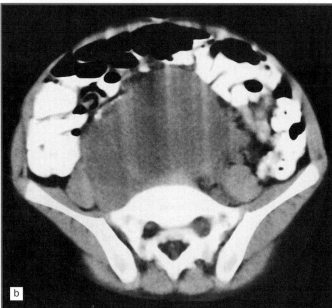

Figure 11.20 *Large intra-abdominal Stage 3 ganglio-neuroblastoma without adverse biological features. (a) CT scan; (b) CT scan 6 months later after a wait-and-watch policy.*

progress has been made. The gold standard chemotherapy remains regimens such as OPEC or PE CADO.

Role of surgery

Initial tumour biopsy is now widely used to document tumour biology, although at present this has little influence on management of Stage 4 disease. Both N-*myc* amplified and non-amplified tumours do relatively poorly. There is debate regarding the value of surgical excision following chemotherapy. In most patients, disease recurs at a distant site and the potential benefit of attempting to resect residual primary tumour remains unclear. These operations are

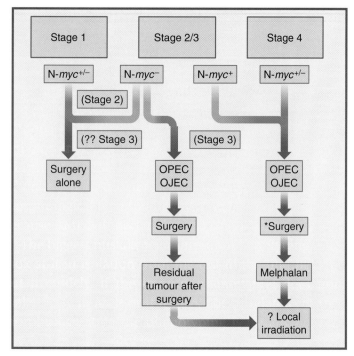

Figure 11.21 *Algorithm for the management of neuroblastoma based on N-*myc* status. *See Figure 11.22.*

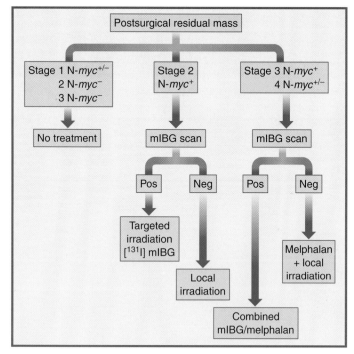

Figure 11.22 *Algorithm for the management of residual tumour mass after surgery and/or chemotherapy.*

often difficult, taking several hours and are not without potential morbidity. It seems logical, however, to apply the same philosophy as used for other childhood tumours and remove the primary tumour where possible, hoping that improvements in chemotherapy will eventually reduce the likelihood of distant recurrence, at which time primary control will emerge as a more important factor.

Role of megatherapy

One study, ENSG 1, has evaluated the role of consolidation of complete or partial remission with a single course of high-dose melphalan using unpurged autologous bone marrow rescue. There is continued debate about this strategy and a range of regimens have been used (Box 11.2). It has been suggested that prolonged chemotherapy may be of value, but this is not of proven benefit.

As in Stage 3 disease, the role of radiotherapy to primary tumour following chemotherapy is unproved. Intraoperative radiotherapy and mIBG therapy have both been used. In general, similar guidelines should be applied to primary tumour for both Stage 3 and Stage 4 disease although this may be guided by tumour biology.

Box 11.2 High-dose therapy regimens in neuroblastoma

Melphalan

Doxorubicin/VM26/melphalan

Vincristine/TBI/melphalan

Carboplatin/etoposide/melphalan

Busulphan/cyclophosphamide/melphalan

Double graft:

VM26/melphalan and busulphan/cyclophosphamide

VM26/cisplatin/carmustine and

vincristine/melphalan/TBI

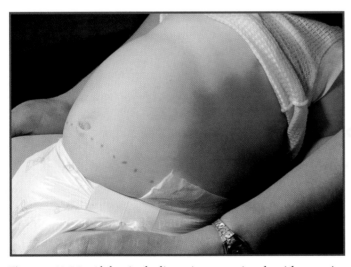

Figure 11.23 *Abdominal distention associated with massive hepatomegaly in a well infant with Stage 4S neuroblastoma.*

Stage 4S disease

The most important aspect of treating patients with Stage 4S disease is to tailor treatment to the general condition of the child (Fig. 11.23). Tumour bulk or extent is of no significance in itself, provided the child is well. Overall, an initial conservative wait-and-see policy is appropriate for all patients. A step-by-step strategy involving the introduction of simple chemotherapy or low-dose local radiotherapy progressing to more intensive chemotherapy is outlined in Figure 11.24.

A small percentage of these tumours will be N-*myc*-positive, and it now seems clear that these patients do badly and should receive more intensive chemotherapy, comparable to that used for Stage 4 disease.

Policies regarding resection of primary tumours vary. It seems illogical to put the child through laparotomy to remove a small calcified primary tumour when there is still evidence of hepatic disease. A recent consensus has recommended that, if after 12 months all distant disease has cleared and the primary tumour is still detectable, then it should be removed.

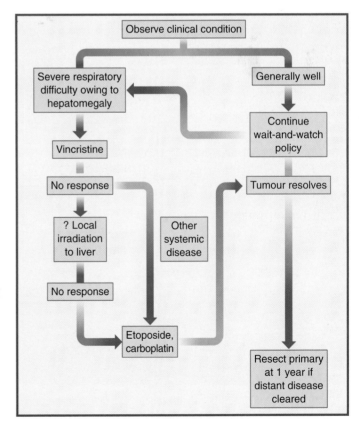

Figure 11.24 *Algorithm for the management of infants with Stage 4S disease.*

Late recurrences associated with residual primary tumour have been observed. Unfortunately, many studies purporting to demonstrate a benefit for surgery have included attempted primary resection at diagnosis. This is wholly unjustified and will increase patient morbidity.

Managing recurrent disease

A small number of patients will fail to respond to primary chemotherapy (Figs. 11.25 and 11.26). As with other tumours, this is the worst subgroup and cure is unlikely. Response at primary site may, however, be slow, and evaluation of distant metastases is more important with regard to deciding that the tumour is chemorefractory. In tumours without N-*myc* amplification second-line chemotherapy should be introduced, although more investigational regimens may be appropriate. The suggested policy for relapsed tumours depending on initial stage is shown in Figure 11.27.

Role of differentiating agents

Tumour differentiation is undoubtedly produced by *cis*-retinoic acid *in vitro*, and this has also been described *in vivo*. The ENSG 4 study randomises between retinoic acid and placebo in patients with high-risk disease who are in complete remission; the outcome at present is unknown.

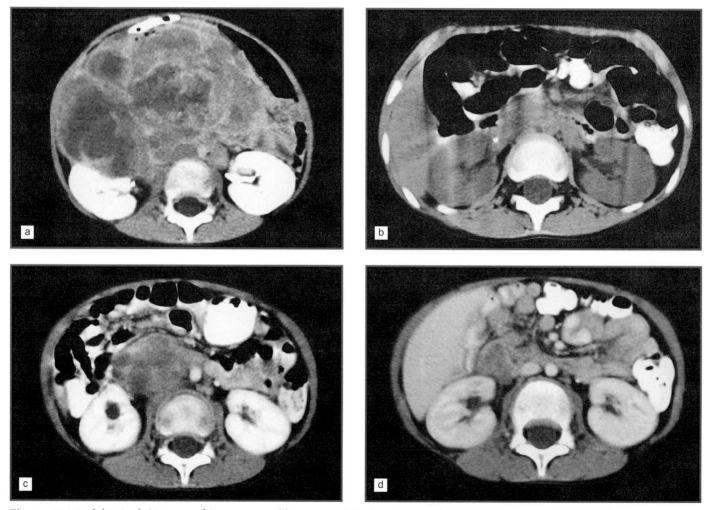

Figure 11.25 *Abdominal CT scans of Stage 3 neuroblastoma with biology typical of poor prognosis. (a) At presentation; (b) following seven courses of OPEC/OJEC; (c) despite this good response, surgery was incomplete and although local irradiation was given, there was a local recurrence within 12 months; (d) second-line therapy with CADO produced an excellent second response. Despite consolidation with high-dose chemotherapy, there was a subsequent relapse.*

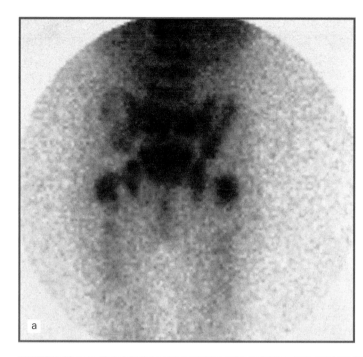

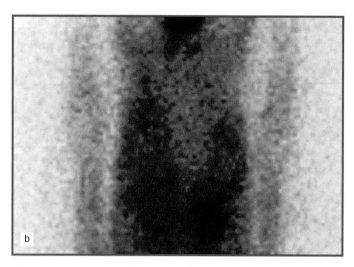

Figure 11.26 *Neuroblastoma refractory to OPEC/OJEC. (a) mIBG scanning; (b) scanning after treatment with etoposide and high-dose cyclosporin A showed an excellent response with no skeletal uptake. Following this, consolidation with high-dose melphalan and PBSC rescue was given.*

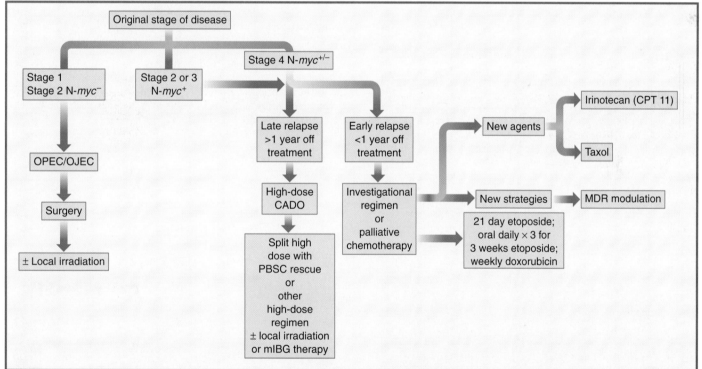

Figure 11.27 *Algorithm for the management of patients with recurrent neuroblastoma.*

Summary

Strategies in neuroblastoma for accurately staging disease and linking biological characteristics with treatment and prognosis are still being developed. Some potential therapies that may be of use in the future are listed in Box 11.3.

Box 11.3 Future strategies in neuroblastoma

Drug-resistance modulation, e.g. PSC 833

Pulsed high-dose therapy with PBSC rescue

Up-front mIBG therapy

New differentiating agents, e.g 9-*cis*-retinoic acid

Vaccine therapy: autologous or allogeneic tumour

Immunotherapy, e.g interleukin-2 after autograft

Further reading

Brodeur, G.M., Pritchard, J., Berthold, F. *et al.* (1993) Revisions of the international criteria for neuroblastoma diagnosis, staging, and response to treatment. *Journal of Clinical Oncology* 11: 1466–1477.

Caron, H., Van Sluis, P.D., de Kraker, J. *et al.* (1996) Allelic loss of chromosome 1p as a predictor of unfavourable outcome in patients with neuroblastoma. *New England Journal of Medicine* 334: 225–230.

Chan, H.S.L., Haddad, G., Thorner, P.S. *et al.* (1991) P-glycoprotein expression as a predictor of the outcome of therapy of neuroblastoma. *New England Journal of Medicine* 325: 1608–1614.

Combaret, V., Gross, N., Lasset, C. *et al.* (1996) Clinical relevance of CD44 cell-surface expression and N-*myc* gene amplification in a multicentric analysis of 121 pediatric neuroblastomas. *Journal of Clinical Oncology* 14: 25–34.

Coze, C., Hartmann, O., Michon, J. *et al.* (1997) NB87 induction protocol for stage 4 neuroblastoma in children over 1 year of age: a report from the French Society of Pediatric Oncology. *Journal of Clinical Oncology* 15: 3433–3440.

DeBernardi, B., Conte, M., Mancini, A. *et al.* (1995) Localized resectable neuroblastoma: results of the second study of the Italian Cooperative Group for Neuroblastoma. *Journal of Clinical Oncology* 13: 884–893.

De Kraker, J., Hoefnagel, C.A., Caron, H. *et al.* (1995) First line targeted radiotherapy, a new concept in the treatment of advanced stage neuroblastoma. *European Journal of Cancer* 31A: 600–602.

Kogner, P., Barbany, G., Dominici, C. *et al.* (1993) Coexpression of messenger RNA for TRK protocogene and low-affinity nerve growth factor receptor in neuroblastoma with favourable prognosis. *Cancer Research* 53: 2044–2050.

Kushner, B.H., Cheung, N.-K.V., LaQuaglia, M.P. *et al.* (1996) Survival from locally invasive or widespread neuroblastoma without cytotoxic therapy. *Journal of Clinical Oncology* 14: 373–381.

Kushner, B.H., O'Reily, R.J., Mandell, L.R. *et al.* (1991) Myeloablative combination without total body irradiation for neuroblastoma. *Journal of Clinical Oncology* 9: 274–279.

Lashford, L.S., Lewis, I.J., Fielding, S.L. *et al.* (1992). A phase I/II study of ^{131}I-mIBG in chemo-resistant neruoblastoma. *Journal of Clinical Oncology* 10: 1889–1896.

Lovat, P.E., Lowis, S.P. and Pearson, A.D.J. (1994) Concentration-dependent effects of 9-*cis*-retinoic acid on neuroblastoma differentiation and proliferation *in vitro*. *Neuroscience Letters*, 182: 29–32.

Matthay, K.K., O'Leary, M.C., Ramsay, N.K. *et al.* (1995) Role of myeloablative therapy in improved outcome for high risk neuroblastoma: reviews of recent Children's Cancer Group results. *European Journal of Cancer* 31A: 572–575.

Matthay, K.K., Sather, H.N., Seeger, R.C. *et al.* (1989) Excellent outcome of stage II neuroblastoma is independent of residual disease and radiation therapy. *Journal of Clinical Oncology* 7: 236–244.

Norris, M.D., Bordow, S. B., Marshall, G.M. *et al.* (1996) Expression of the gene for multidrug resistance-associated protein and outcome in patients with neuroblastoma. *New England Journal of Medicine* 334: 231–238.

Pearson, A.D.J., Craft, A.W., Pinkerton, C.R. *et al.* (1992) High dose rapid schedule chemotherapy for disseminated neuroblastoma. *European Journal of Cancer* 28A: 1654–1659.

Pinkerton, C.R., Pritchard, J., de Kraker, J. *et al.* (1987). ENSG 1 – randomised study of high dose melphalan in neuroblastoma. In *Autologous Bone Marrow Transplantation* (eds K.A. Dicke, G. Spitzer and S. Jagonnoth), University of Texas Press, Texas, pp. 401–405.

Pinkerton, C.R., Zucker, J.M., Hartmann, O. *et al.* (1990) Short duration, high dose, alternating chemotherapy in metastatic neuroblastoma (ENSG 3C induction regimen). *British Journal of Cancer* 62: 319–323.

Rubie, H., Hartmann, O., Michon, J. *et al.* (1997) N-*myc* gene amplification is a major prognostic factor in localized neuroblastoma: results of the French NBL 90 study. *Journal of Clinical Oncology* 15: 1171–1182.

Tsuchida, Y., Yokoyama, J., Kaneko, M. *et al.* (1992) Therapeutic significance of surgery in advanced neuroblastoma: a report from the study group of Japan. *Journal of Pediatric Surgery* 27: 616–622.

CHAPTER 12

Ewing's sarcoma/primitive neuro-ectodermal tumour

C.R. Pinkerton

Introduction

Considerable discussion has taken place in recent years regarding the distinction between Ewing's sarcoma of bone, soft tissue Ewing's, primitive neuro-ectodermal tumour of soft tissue and primitive neuro-ectodermal tumour of bone. All these tumours share the t(11;22) translocation and are likely, therefore, to have a common biological origin. There are, however, some differences in behaviour in relation to both anatomical site and specific pathological features. The debate has been bedevilled by difficulties in standardising terminology. It appears appropriate to regard any tumour within the 'Ewing's family' that has evidence of neural differentiation, either immunohistochemically or on electron microscopy, as a PNET. All others should be called either soft tissue Ewing's sarcoma or Ewing's sarcoma of bone. Intracranial PNETs must not be confused with this group: they are unrelated, and biologically and histologically distinct. Treatment strategies for Ewing's sarcoma are dependent on the site of tumour as much as on the pathology, as will be discussed below.

Initially, the diagnosis of Ewing's sarcoma was essentially one made by exclusion. For Ewing's sarcoma of bone, the main differential diagnoses were small cell osteosarcoma, neuroblastoma, lymphoma or metastatic rhabdomyosarcoma. These would all have immunohistochemical features supportive of the individual diagnosis. More recently, semi-specific antibodies such as MIC-2 or the use of electron microscopy have supported a specific diagnosis of Ewing's sarcoma (Fig. 12.1).

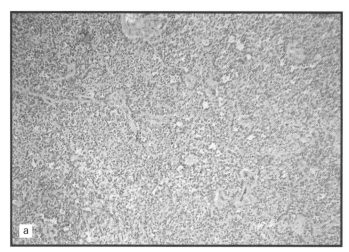

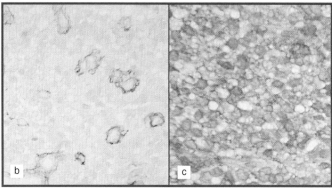

Figure 12.1 *Histopathological features of Ewing's sarcoma. (a) General morphology; (b) NSE positivity; (c) MIC-2 antibody.*

Molecular pathology

The demonstration of the t(11;22) translocation in the majority, if not at all, Ewing's sarcomas has facilitated the classification of this tumour type. There are variations in the transcript produced but to date this has not been clearly shown to correlate with biological behaviour. A range of methods can be used to demonstrate this translocation, including FISH (Fig. 12.2), Southern analysis or RT–PCR. In addition to being of value in confirming diagnosis, cytogenetic studies may have a role to play in detection of minimal disease, either at presentation or following treatment. Ongoing studies are assessing the potential prognostic significance of minimal disease detected only using RT–PCR in patients who would otherwise be staged as non-metastatic using conventional imaging, bone marrow morphology and cytology. Preliminary results have confirmed that a significant number of patients are positive solely with RT–PCR, but to what extent this influences outcome remains unclear.

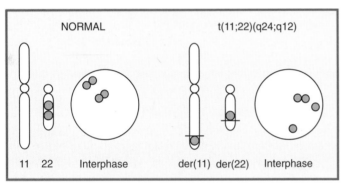

Figure 12.2 *Schematic representation of FISH study of t(11;22), translocation. In the normal cell the probes that flank the site of translocation are positioned close together; in the tumour tissue the red and green signals are separated as a result of the translocation.*

Clinical staging

As for osteosarcoma, a rather crude staging system is used for Ewing's sarcoma of bone. Patients are divided on the basis of the presence or absence of metastases. Other features such as tumour volume, LDH and, perhaps, microscopic response at surgery following primary chemotherapy are all of potential importance and should ultimately be incorporated in a new staging system. Because of improvements in the outcome of this tumour in recent years, it has been difficult to identify clearly independent prognostic factors.

Management

Surgery: when should it be performed and what procedures?

It is logical that complete excision of any expendable bone should be carried out as early as possible following initial chemotherapy (Fig. 12.3). In the case

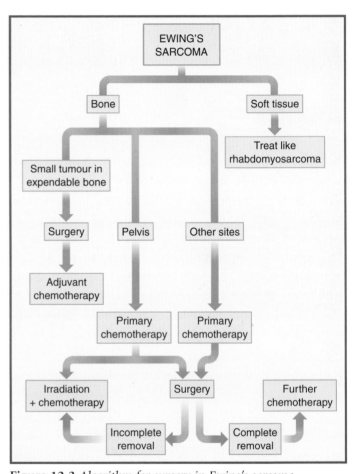

Figure 12.3 *Algorithm for surgery in Ewing's sarcoma.*

of tumours involving digits, initial amputation may be appropriate. In most cases at least four courses of initial chemotherapy are given prior to an attempt at conservative non-mutilating surgery. In some patients, this is comparatively straightforward, for example, those with tumours of a limb or rib (Figs. 12.4–12.6), but for pelvic primaries the situation is more complex (Figs. 12.7–12.10).

In the past, high-dose local radiotherapy was used to avoid amputation, but with the introduction of prosthetic procedures the strategy now resembles that

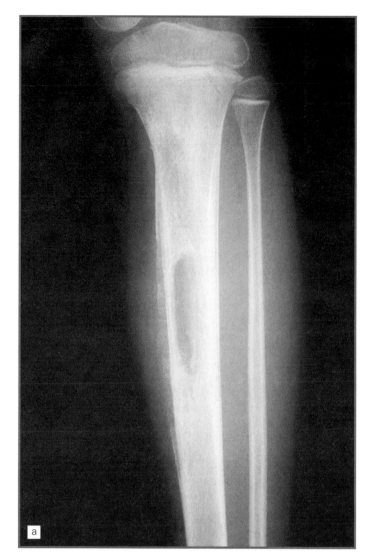
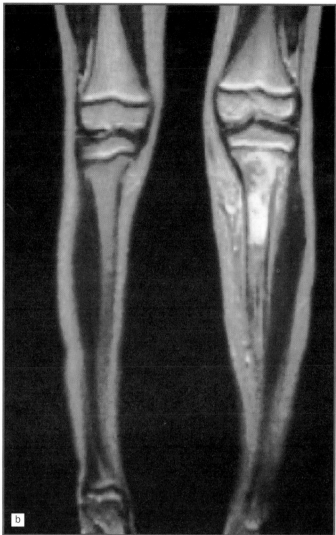

Figure 12.4 *Localised tibial Ewing's sarcoma. (a) Plain X-ray film; (b) MRI scan which demonstrates the extent of soft tissue infiltration. The abnormal signal extends up the medullary cavity on the MR image to a more extensive degree than is apparent on the plain film.*

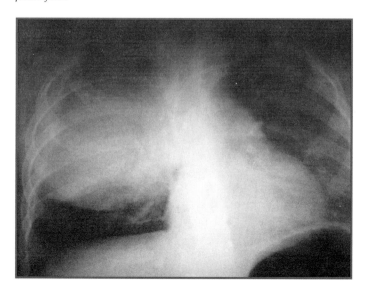

Figure 12.5 *Plain radiograph of rib Ewing's sarcoma with extensive soft tissue involvement; destruction of the rib is evident.*

used for osteogenic sarcoma. In most cases, preoperative chemotherapy will reduce the extent of soft tissue infiltration and enable complete removal of the tumour with an acceptable margin. Macroscopic, or even microscopic, residual disease following surgery is now uncommon. In the case of bulky pelvic tumours, surgery was felt to be inappropriate and technically problematic. It is now possible to use reconstructive surgery for almost all pelvic tumours. The sole exclusion is where the sacro-iliac joint is involved (Fig. 12.9).

Management of residual disease following surgery

To try to maximise the likelihood of local control, radiotherapy is usually used. Doses of 45–65 Gy are

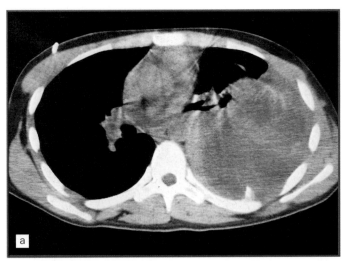
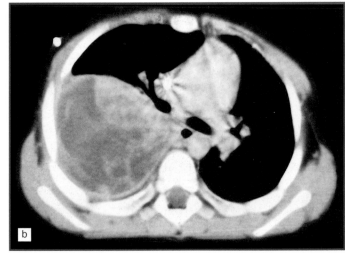

Figure 12.6 *(a and b) Soft tissue Ewing's sarcomas of the chest wall. In (a) a small spicule of bone indicates that this may, in fact, have arisen on the inner surface of the bone. In this patient the plain X-ray image of the rib was normal.*

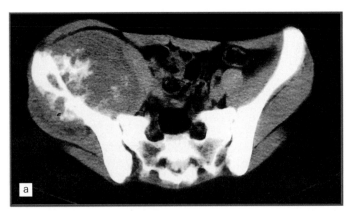
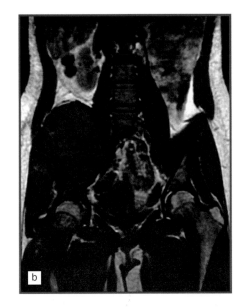

Figure 12.7 *Large pelvic Ewing's sarcoma involving the right iliac bone. (a) CT; (b) MRI.*

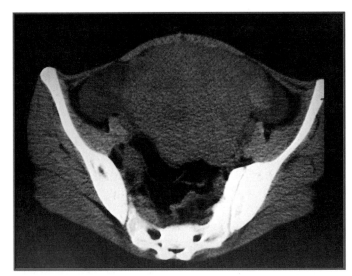
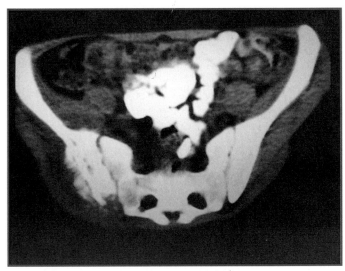

Figure 12.8 *Pelvic Ewing's sarcoma arising in right iliac bone but with a predominant soft tissue component.*

Figure 12.9 *Pelvic Ewing's sarcoma with extensive infiltration across the sacro-iliac joint, thus precluding surgical excision.*

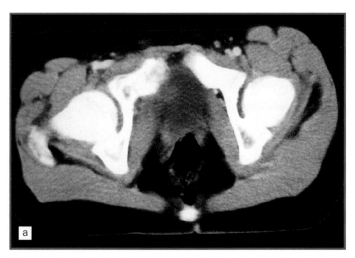 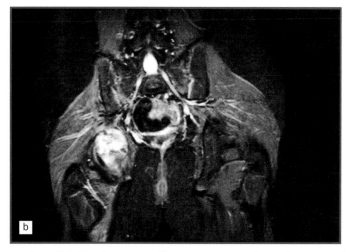

Figure 12.10 *Ewing's sarcoma of the pubic bone. (a) Initial presentation. (b) Despite an excellent response to chemotherapy and apparent complete excision, there was a local recurrence at the distal extent of original surgery.*

used depending on age and site. In the EICESS protocol, the dose of radiotherapy varies depending on the extent of residual active tumour in the resected specimen and 45 Gy is given even in the case of complete clearance where more than 10% of residual active tumour is found. This policy is probably unnecessarily aggressive. A dose of 55 Gy is used for marginal clearance or microscopic residual disease. There is, however, circumstantial evidence from small numbers of patients indicating that continued chemotherapy may be adequate to achieve local control in chemosensitive tumours where microscopic residual disease persists following surgery. In both the EICESS and the UKCCSG studies, these patients were protocol violations, but despite the elective omission of radiotherapy by investigators, local control was achieved. This issue needs to be addressed prospectively with larger numbers. There is obvious reluctance to use irradiation following extensive surgery and insertion of prostheses, in addition to the usual concern about the risk of radiation-induced tumours.

Types of chemotherapy

There is little doubt that escalation of the dose of alkylating agent and anthracycline has significantly improved the outcome in Ewing's sarcoma. Dose escalation of cyclophosphamide from 0.6 to 1.5 g/m^2 or above, or the replacement of cyclophosphamide by 6–9 g/m^2 ifosfamide has generally been combined with an increase in the dose of anthracycline up to 75–90

mg/m^2. It seems likely that 1.5–2 g/m^2 cyclophosphamide is comparable to 5–6 g/m^2 ifosfamide, but there are few data that indicate that a dose of 9 g/m^2 ifosfamide is superior to 6 g/m^2. It is difficult to separate the improved efficacy of chemotherapy from a likely improvement owing to more radical surgery. The additional potential benefit of adding etoposide to the basic IVAAd (ifosfamide, vincristine, actinomycin, doxorubicin) regimen is being addressed by the current EICESS/UKCCSG protocol. A randomised trial from the CCG has demonstrated that the addition of ifosfamide plus etoposide significantly improved the outcome in non-metastatic Ewing's sarcoma. Retrospective dose-intensity analyses have indicated that doxorubicin is the single most important agent and actinomycin D may be not only less active but, when given at the expense of the dose of anthracycline, may in fact be detrimental. The S.F.O.P. group have expressed concern about the potential enhancement of anthracycline cardiac toxicity when it is combined with ifosfamide and have recommended the St Jude protocol from the mid-1980s, which combines prolonged oral scheduling of cyclophosphamide with a policy of continuing actinomycin D throughout local radiotherapy.

Management of children with distant metastases remains frustrating, and the introduction of dose-intense regimens followed by myeloablative chemoradiotherapy has to date had little impact on outcome. Unlike in osteogenic sarcoma, metastatectomy for lung disease has little role to play and it seems likely that the dose achieved by bilateral lung irradiation is unlikely to significantly contribute to improved outcome. Local irradiation of multiple bony metastases may be of some palliative benefit, but the outcome in patients with either bone or bone marrow disease is grim and these patients should be entered onto investigational protocols (Fig. 12.11).

Management of soft tissue Ewing's sarcoma

Soft tissue Ewing's sarcoma or PNET are biologically similar to bony Ewing's sarcoma and it seems likely that they share a similar chemosensitivity profile (Figs. 12.12–12.14). Data from the IRS have shown that treatment using VAC without doxorubicin produces results comparable to that for rhabdomyosarcoma and it seems unlikely that anthracyclines significantly increase relapse-free survival for these patients. Bone involvement may require more aggressive treatment but with soft tissue tumours a less intensive chemotherapy protocol may be adequate, thus avoiding the late effects of anthracyclines. The current SIOP recommendation is that these patients should be

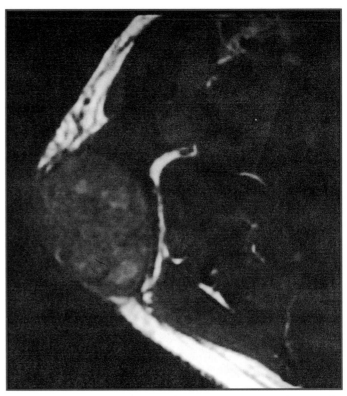

Figure 12.12 *Soft tissue Ewing's sarcoma involving the scapular region.*

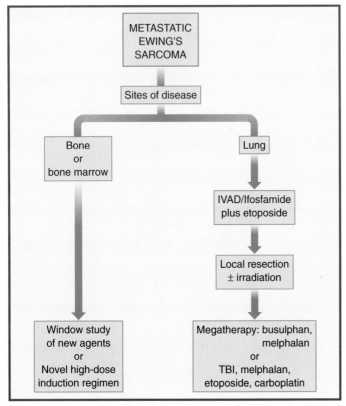

Figure 12.11 *Algorithm for treatment of metastatic Ewing's sarcoma.*

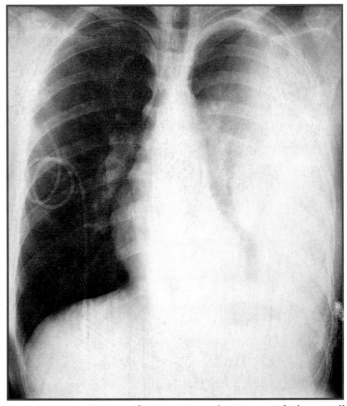

Figure 12.13 *Large soft tissue Ewing's tumour of chest wall (Askin tumour).*

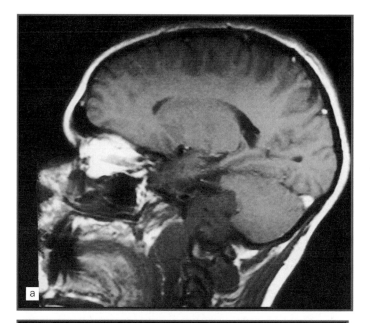

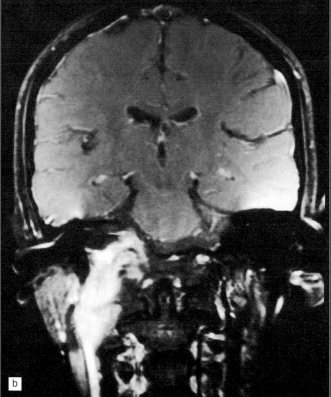

Figure 12.14 *MRI scans, (a) lateral, (b) anteroposterior, of a soft tissue Ewing's sarcoma involving the base of the skull and the paravertebral region.*

treated on the IVA protocol, as for rhabdomyosarcoma. Analysis of patients treated in this way is awaited and should the outcome be poorer than expected, then it would be appropriate to intensify therapy with an IVAd-based protocol.

Treatment duration

Ewing's sarcoma is the only solid tumour in paediatrics where treatment is prolonged to at least a year. The logic for this is unclear. Shorter, more dose-intensive regimens have been used but the numbers of patients have always been small. There remains a general reluctance to consider more than a minimal reduction in duration, i.e. the current EICESS protocol has been reduced to around 10 months.

Role of local irradiation

For the unresectable tumour, high-dose irradiation (50–60 Gy) remains the mainstay of local treatment. This should be used relatively early in treatment, as the degree of tumour reduction does not generally alter the size of the radiation field. Most radiotherapists would plan the radiation field on the initial tumour bulk and, therefore, there is little to be gained from prolonged pre-radiotherapy chemotherapy. Novel schedules of irradiation are under evaluation, including the use of hyper-fractionation and split regimens given simultaneously with dose-intensive chemotherapy.

Outcome of recurrent disease

Very few children with recurrent disease will be long-term survivors (Fig. 12.15). A small number with original small-bulk disease who did not receive radiotherapy and have a local relapse may be salvaged by radical surgery, i.e. amputation, with second-line adjuvant chemotherapy. There are few effective second-line chemotherapy regimens. The most effective appears to be ifosfamide/etoposide, particularly in patients who have been previously treated with standard dose cyclophosphamide. Cisplatin/etoposide has also been used, but both cisplatin and carboplatin as single agents have only limited activity in Ewing's sarcoma. In this situation, it is appropriate to consider six courses of standard chemotherapy and consolidate remission with an escalation of alkylating agent-based regimens, such as those shown in Box 12.1. Figure 12.16 outlines a strategy for relapsed Ewing's sarcoma.

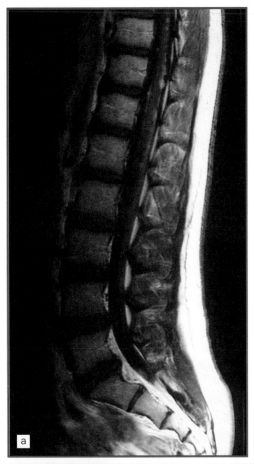

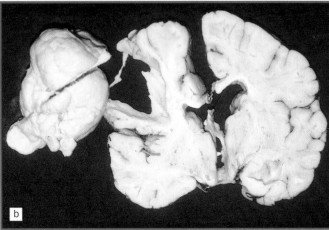

Figure 12.15 *Recurrent PNET. (a) Intraspinal metastases; (b) intracerebral metastasis.*

Box 12.1 High-dose regimens in Ewing's sarcoma

Melphalan

Vincristine/melphalan/TBI

Busulphan/melphalan ± thiotepa

Melphalan/etoposide/carboplatin + TBI

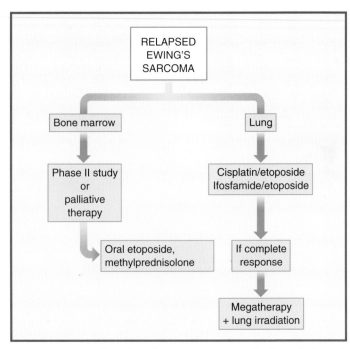

Figure 12.16 *Algorithm for management of relapsed Ewing's sarcoma.*

Further reading

Ambros, I.M., Ambros, P.F., Strehl, S. *et al.* (1990) MIC2 is a specific marker for Ewing's sarcoma and peripheral primitive neuroectodermal tumours. Evidence for a common histogenesis of neuroectodermal tumors from MIC2 expression and specific chromosome aberration. *Cancer* 67: 1886–1893.

Atra, A., Whelan, J.S., Calvagna, V., Shankar, A.G. *et al.* (1997) High-dose busulphan/melphalan with autologous stem cell rescue in Ewing's sarcoma. *Bone Marrow Transplant* 20: 843–846.

Burdach, S., Jurgens, H., Peters, C. *et al.* (1993) Myeloablative radiochemotherapy and hematopoietic stem-cell rescue in poor-prognosis Ewing's sarcoma. *Journal of Clinical Oncology* 11: 1482–1488.

Craft, A.W., Cotterill, S.J., Bullimore, J.A. *et al.* (1997) Long-term results from the first UKCCSG Ewing's tumour Study (ET-1). *European Journal of Cancer* 33: 1061–1069.

Craft, A.W., Cotterill, S. and Imeson, J. (1993) Improvement in survival for Ewing's sarcoma by substitution of ifosfamide for cyclophosphamide. A UKCCSG study. *American Journal of Pediatric Hematology and Oncology* 15 (Suppl. A): 31–35.

Dehner, L.P. (1994) Neuroepithelioma (primitive neuroectodermal tumor) and Ewing's sarcoma. At least a partial consensus. *Archives in Pathology and Laboratory Medicine* 118: 606–607.

Dunst, J., Jurgens, H., Sauer, R. *et al.* (1995) Radiation therapy in Ewing's sarcoma: an update of the CESS 86 trial. *International Journal of Radiation Oncology, Biology and Physics* 32: 919–930.

Kushner, B.H., Meyers, P.A., Gerald, W.L. *et al.* (1995) Very-high-dose short-term chemotherapy for poor-risk peripheral primitive neuroectodermal tumors, including Ewing's sarcoma, in children and young adults. *Journal of Clinical Oncology* 13: 2796–2804.

Ladenstein, R., Lasset, C., Pinkerton, R. *et al.* (1995) Impact of megatherapy in children with high-risk Ewing's tumours in complete remission: a report from the EBMT Solid Tumour Registry. *Bone Marrow Transplant* 15: 697–705.

Navarro, S., Cavazzana, A.O., Llombart-Bosch, A. and Triche, T.J. (1994) Comparison of Ewing's sarcoma of bone and peripheral neuroepithelioma. *Archives in Pathology and Laboratory Medicine* 118: 608–615.

Roessener, A., Ueda, K., Bockhorn-Dworniczak, B. *et al.* (1993) Prognostic implication of immunodetection of P glycoprotein in Ewing's sarcoma. *Journal of Cancer Research and Clinical Oncology* 119: 185–189.

West, D.C., Grier, H.E., Swallow, M.M. *et al.* (1997) Detection of circulating tumor cells in patients with Ewing's sarcoma and peripheral primitive neuroectodermal tumor. *Journal of Clinical Oncology* 15: 583–588.

CHAPTER 13

Osteogenic sarcoma

C.R. Pinkerton

Introduction

In the past some patients with osteogenic sarcoma were cured by radical surgery, i.e. amputation, but the introduction of adjuvant chemotherapy post-operatively improved progression-free survival and subsequently facilitated the use of conservative surgery. In this tumour, more than almost any other, close co-ordination between experienced orthopaedic surgeons and oncologists is essential to optimise both the time of surgery and the nature of tumour resection. In this way, cure may be achieved with limited long-term disability.

A plain X-ray of a painful bone or site of bony swelling may produce pathognomonic features of osteosarcoma (Figs. 13.1 and 13.2). CT scanning will clarify the extent of bony disease, and to some extent the soft tissue infiltration, but MRI is necessary to define most clearly the extent of abnormal tissue adjacent to the primary destructive bone lesion (Figs. 13.3 and 13.4). Imaging may classify tumours into the less common periosteal or paraosteal subtypes, which is of prognostic significance. Paraosteal tumours are invariably low grade, for which surgery alone is curative; in most cases, the normal bone adjacent to the tumour can remain intact without the need for radical resection. For periosteal tumours, surgery alone is probably sufficient but needs to be more radical in order to guarantee local control.

A number of histological subtypes of osteogenic sarcoma have been described (Table 13.1), but with current treatment strategies the prognostic implications of these are unclear. In the past

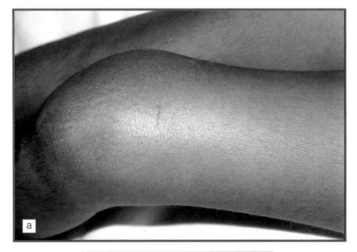

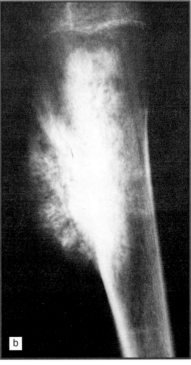

Figure 13.1 *Osteosarcoma. (a) Presenting as swelling of the knee; (b) plain X-ray film shows typical 'sunburst' appearance.*

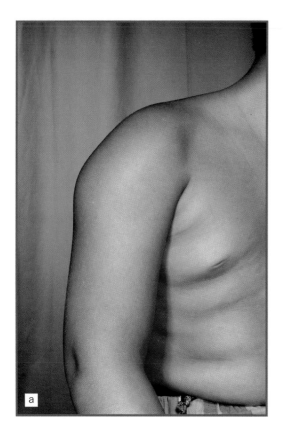

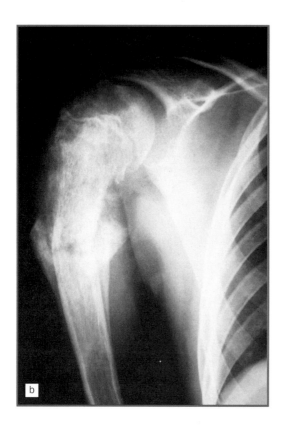

Figure 13.2 *Osteosarcoma of upper humerus. (a) Presenting with painful swelling; (b) plain X-ray film shows a typical calcified soft tissue mass with pathological fracture.*

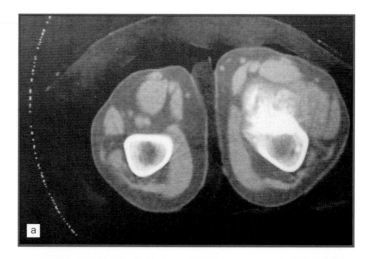

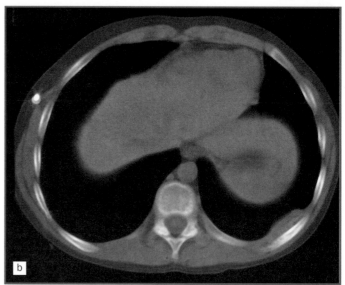

Figure 13.3 *CT scan in osteosarcoma. (a) Scan shows the extent of soft tissue infiltration adjacent to the osteosarcoma; (b) a bony metastasis in a rib plus soft tissue infiltration.*

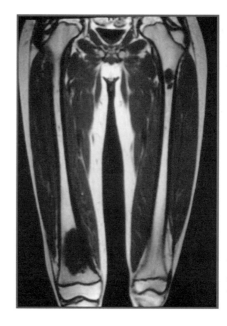

Figure 13.4 *MRI scan shows primary lesion plus single bony metastasis in contralateral upper femur.*

Table 13.1 Histological patterns of osteosarcoma	
Type	Incidence (%)
Osteoblastic	78
Chondroblastic	4
Fibroblastic	4
Malignant fibrous histiocytoma-like	<1
Giant cell-rich	<1
Telangiectatic	<1
Low-grade intraosseous	<1
Small cell	<1
Juxtacortical	
Paraosteal	<1
Periosteal	<1

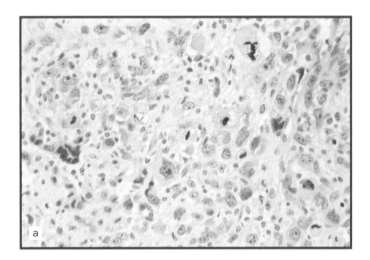

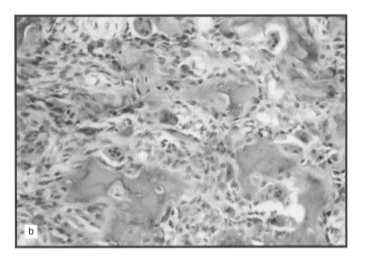

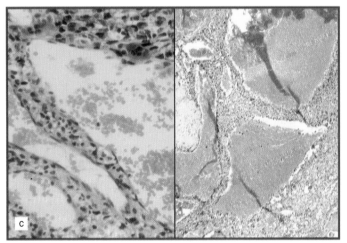

Figure 13.5 *Pathological features of osteogenic sarcoma. (a) Undifferentiated; (b) osteoblastic; (c) telangiectatic.*

telangiectatic osteosarcoma and undifferentiated small cell osteosarcoma were said to have a higher risk of metastatic relapse (Fig. 13.5).

Because of the trend towards attempting conservative sparing surgery, a limited initial biopsy is to be encouraged. Many specialist orthopaedic centres would now recommend a percutaneous trephine biopsy. The core biopsy obtained in this way may be adequate for a confident histological diagnosis to be made. A small incision and limited open biopsy is an alternative, but there is no excuse for a large incision and extensive open-biopsy procedure. This will risk local contamination of soft tissue and may compromise subsequent surgery. In the event of an extensive open biopsy, the original scar must be excised in its entirety at the time of later definitive surgery, which may limit the skin cover available postoperatively. Moreover, skin contamination with tumour at the time of initial biopsy may increase the risk of local failure following conservative surgery.

Role of molecular pathology

Even with minimal biopsy, sufficient tissue should be obtained for the range of molecular pathology studies now being performed on most other paediatric cancers. Ploidy has been suggested as a potential prognostic indicator, with near diploid tumours doing less well. Similarly, expression of P-glycoprotein, reflecting MDR-1 overexpression, was also reported to have a higher failure rate. Both these require to be confirmed in larger studies where standard chemotherapy has been used.

Staging

In the absence of other clinical prognostic factors, osteogenic sarcoma is generally classified as either localised or metastatic. A number of studies have attempted to assess the independent adverse prognostic impact of tumour bulk, LDH and response to initial preoperative chemotherapy, but at present there is no standardised staging system that incorporates any of these parameters.

Lung metastases may be apparent on chest radiographs (Fig. 13.6) but CT scanning is regarded as the standard method of detecting small metastases. The findings of MRI and CT scans do not necessarily overlap and in some tumours both modalities may be desirable. The extent of intramedullary disease is shown more clearly on MRI, although bony involvement may be better shown with CT. Similarly, soft tissue infiltration is usually more extensive on MRI, although it is impossible to distinguish to what extent some of this abnormal signal is related to tumour oedema rather than tumour.

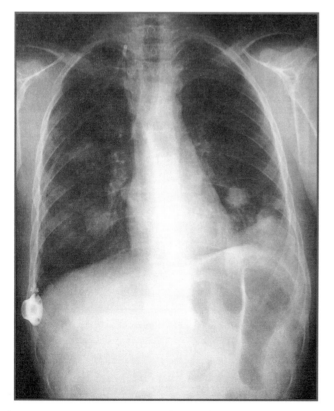

Figure 13.6 *Osteosarcoma. A plain radiograph showing obvious multiple bilateral metastases.*

Technetium bone scan is a standard procedure as part of initial staging in order to exclude the unusual polyostotic variant or discreet bony secondaries.

Preoperative chemotherapy

Since the first demonstration by the POG group of a disease-free survival advantage where adjuvant chemotherapy was used following amputation, and the subsequent introduction of preoperative chemotherapy to facilitate conservative surgery, the latter has become standard practice. There are now few contraindications to the use of preoperative chemotherapy; ones that do occur are:

- compound fracture with extensive soft tissue contamination
- necrotic ulcerated tumour
- young child with femoral or tibial tumour, e.g. less than 8 years of age.

Considerable debate continues regarding the optimal chemotherapy to be given either preoperatively or as an adjuvant following amputation. The original multidrug Rosen regimen has been replicated by the SFOP group, with encouraging results. However, randomised comparison of a Rosen or Rosen-type regimen with the simpler doxorubicin/cisplatin regimen by the EORTC/MRC/UKCCSG indicates that multiagent regimens may not be required. At present in the UK, doxorubicin/cisplatin is the standard treatment for non-metastatic patients. There is, however, an argument against this with regard to toxicity. If comparable results may be obtained with a high-dose methotrexate-based regimen, then this may be preferable on the grounds of fewer late sequelae.

Type of surgery and its timing

In patients where there has been minimal soft tissue infiltration at presentation, or where there has been a clear response of soft tissue involvement with primary chemotherapy, conservative limb-sparing surgery should be attempted (Figs. 13.7 and 13.8). It is now relatively unusual for an amputation to be required following preoperative chemotherapy. In general, surgery is arranged after 6–9 weeks of chemotherapy.

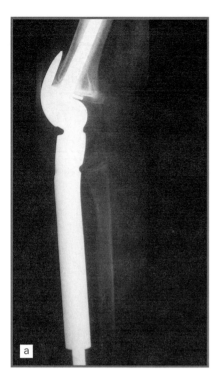
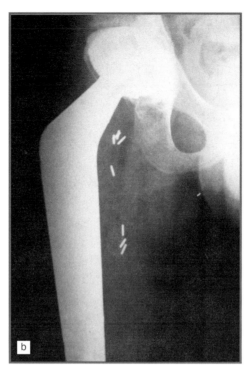
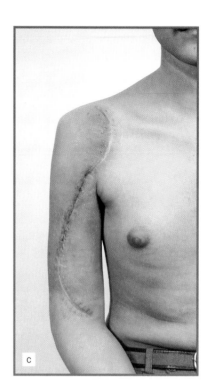

Figure 13.7 *Prosthetic joints for (a) knee; (b) hip; and (c) shoulder.*

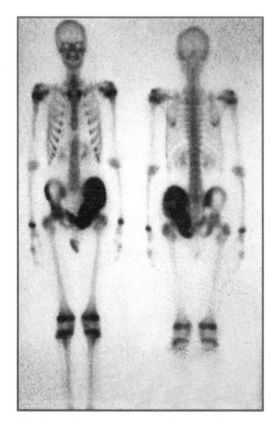

Figure 13.8 *Large iliac osteosarcoma shown on bone scan. In this case, there was little shrinkage with chemotherapy but limb-sparing surgery involving hemipelvectomy and fibula graft reconstruction was feasible. In this situation high dose local irradiation may be indicated as an alternative.*

This requires careful planning, as a complex prosthesis for knee, elbow or shoulder may be required to be individually constructed and surgery must be timed to avoid periods of myelosuppression. Moreover, it is desirable that chemotherapy is restarted as soon as possible following surgery in order to avoid a long gap without treatment.

Should treatment be modified in relation to response? A number of different classifications have been devised to define tumour response to chemotherapy (Table 13.2). In general, the degree of necrosis is an independent prognostic factor. The main debate centres around whether a change in chemotherapy for poor responders can improve the ultimate outcome. The original studies by Rosen suggested that a change from a high-dose methotrexate-based protocol to one containing doxorubicin and cisplatin did improve outcome, but this has not been the case in most other studies. It seems likely that the tumours that initially respond poorly are biologically aggressive and inherently chemoresistant, and alternative novel strategies are required for this group.

Grade	Effect
I	Little or no effect identified
II	Areas of acellular tumour osteoid, necrotic and/or fibrotic material attributable to the effect of chemotherapy, with other areas of histologically viable tumour
III	Predominant areas of acellular tumour osteoid, necrotic and/or fibrotic material attributable to the effect of chemotherapy, with only scattered foci of histologically viable tumour cells identified
IV	No histological evidence of viable tumour identified within the entire specimen

Table 13.2 Histological grading of the effect of preoperative chemotherapy on primary osteosarcoma

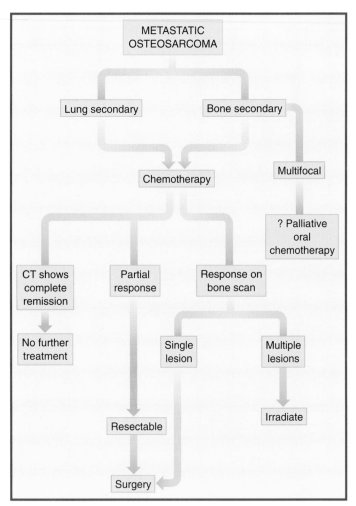

Figure 13.9 *Algorithm for management of metastatic osteosarcoma.*

Management of metastatic disease

If chest X-ray shows metastases, the CT will reveal twice the number and at surgery double the number shown on CT will be found. Predicting the likelihood of complete surgical resection is, therefore, difficult. With bilateral lesions, metastatectomy may be done in two stages or via a sternal split single-step procedure. In general, residual lung metastases at the end of chemotherapy are resected, although to what extent this contributes to long-term survival is unclear. Intensive chemotherapy protocols introducing drugs such as ifosfamide or high-dose cyclophosphamide have been evaluated but data are limited. Overall, the results for treatment of primary metastatic disease remain very disappointing. In the case of polyostotic or bone metastases, the outcome is grim. There are very few long-term survivors and one might question the use of very intensive high-morbidity chemotherapy in this group of patients. The role of local radiotherapy for bone metastases is debatable, and some would argue that this should be restricted to a palliative role (Fig. 13.9).

Management of relapse

As with most tumours, management of relapse will depend on the initial stage and nature of primary chemotherapy. A potential strategy is outlined in Figure 13.10.

Novel treatment strategies

There has been little evidence of striking activity from newer chemotherapy agents such as the taxanes or topo-isomerase I inhibitors, but there is currently interest in immunomodulation or vaccines. Liposmal MTP-PE, a derivative of BCG, has been used as an immunostimulant. The observation that the cell line used to develop an anti-idiotype vaccine for colon carcinoma originated from a patient with osteogenic sarcoma has now been taken forward into early trials of this vaccine in osteosarcoma.

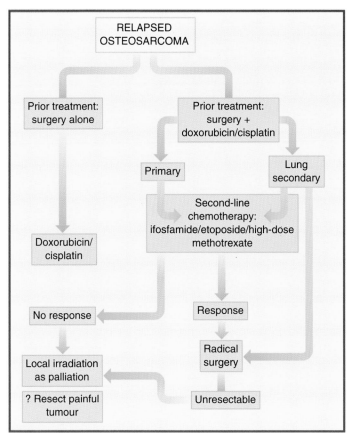

Figure 13.10 *Algorithm for the management of relapsed osteosarcoma.*

Further reading

Bramwell, V.H.C., Burgers, M., Sneath, R. *et al.* (1992) A comparison of two short intensive adjuvant chemotherapy regimens in operable osteosarcoma of limbs in children and young adults: the first study of the European Osteosarcoma Intergroup. *Journal of Clinical Oncology* 10: 1579–1591.

Davis, A.M., Bell, R.S. and Goodwin, P.J. (1994) Prognostic factors in osteosarcoma: a critical review. *Journal of Clinical Oncology* 12: 1423–1431.

Graf, N., Winkler, K., Betlemovic, M. *et al.* (1994) Methotrexate pharmacokinetics and prognosis in osteosarcoma. *Journal of Clinical Oncology* 12: 1443–1451.

Holscher, H.C., Bloem, J. L., van-der-Woude, H.J. *et al.* (1995) Can MRI predict the histopathological response in patients with osteosarcoma after the first cycle of chemotherapy? *Clinical Radiology* 50: 384–390.

Ornadel, D., Souhami, R. L., Whelan, J. *et al.* (1994) Doxorubicin and cisplatin with granulocyte colony-stimulating factor as adjuvant chemotherapy for osteosarcoma: phase II trial of the European Osteosarcoma Intergroup. *Journal of Clinical Oncology* 12: 1842–1848.

Picci, P., Sangiorgi, L., Rougraff, G.T. *et al.* (1994) Relationship of chemotherapy-induced necrosis and surgical margins to local recurrence in osteosarcoma. *Journal of Clinical Oncology* 12: 2699–2705.

Tabone, M., Kalifa, C., Rodary, C. *et al.* (1994) Osteosarcoma recurrence in pediatric patients previously treated with intensive chemotherapy. *Journal of Clinical Oncology* 12: 2614–2620.

Wellings, R.M., Davies, A.M., Pynsent, P.B. *et al.* (1994) The value of computed tomographic measurements in osteosarcoma as a predictor of response to adjuvant chemotherapy. *Clinical Radiology* 49: 19–23.

Winkler, K., Bielack, S., Delling, G. *et al.* (1990) Effect of intraarterial versus intravenous cisplatin in addition to systemic doxorubicin, high-dose methotrexate, and ifosfamide on histologic tumor response in osteosarcoma (Study COSS-86). *Cancer* 66: 1703–1710.

Wunder, J.S., Bell, R.S., Wold, L. and Andrulis, I.L. (1993) Expression of the multidrug resistance gene in osteosarcoma: a pilot study. *Journal of Orthopedic Research* 11: 396–403.

CHAPTER 14
Wilms tumour

C.R. Pinkerton

Introduction

Wilms tumour was the first childhood cancer to be treated with effective chemotherapy. Although the current cure rate is amongst the highest for any childhood cancer, management is not without continuing controversy. This centres around the most appropriate strategy, including both chemotherapy and radiotherapy, that will maintain high cure rates but avoid undesirable late sequelae.

Need for diagnostic biopsy

One of the major controversies is the use of preoperative chemotherapy prior to definitive surgery. The European (SIOP) approach has been to give chemotherapy with vincristine and actinomycin D (prior to this it involved the use of preoperative irradiation). By comparison, in America (North American National Wilms Tumor Study: NWTS) definitive resection is attempted at the time of initial diagnosis. In the UK (UKCCSG) when tumours were judged to be probably inoperable, trucut or limited open biopsy was performed to confirm the diagnosis and three-drug (i.e. more intensive) chemotherapy was administered prior to any attempted surgery. When the tumour was judged to be operable, then primary surgery was done and subsequent chemotherapy depended on the surgical staging, as with the NWTS. In the SIOP studies, tumour biopsy was not mandatory. Indeed, it has been suggested that the use of trucut

biopsies may increase the risk of recurrent disease within the soft tissue track made by the biopsy instrument. There are anecdotal reports of recurrence at this site, but the efficacy of systemic chemotherapy makes it most unlikely that any small number of tumours seeding at the site of biopsy would subsequently produce a local recurrence in the absence of chemoresistant disease elsewhere.

The SIOP group has argued that preoperative chemotherapy reduces the risk of tumour spillage and will increase the likelihood of complete resection or negative nodes at the time of surgery. Consequently, a higher percentage avoid the use of a three-drug regimen, and in particular the use of an anthracycline. It is clear that the percentage of Stage I and II patients is higher where preoperative chemotherapy is used, and at present there is little evidence to suggest that the overall relapse-free survival is adversely affected by such therapeutic downstaging. Not performing a routine biopsy results in up to a 2–4% false diagnosis rate where imaging and supplementary studies, such as urinary catecholamines, are relied on for the diagnosis. Intrarenal neuroblastoma, rhabdoid tumour of kidney, renal carcinoma or benign cystic lesions are the most common incorrect diagnoses.

Is it mandatory to perform urinary catecholamines prior to initial surgery? If the diagnosis is neuroblastoma, potentially severe complications may arise owing to catecholamine-related hypertension during any surgical procedure. If catecholamine results can be obtained rapidly then it is logical to await the results, but as careful preoperative imaging will rule out the majority of neuroblastoma, it is probably not necessary to wait a number of days for a catecholamine result before proceeding with diagnostic biopsy or definitive resection.

Pathology

Pathological subtypes

It has become clear that some pathological subtypes previously classified under the broad heading of 'unfavourable-history' nephroblastoma are biologically different entities and should probably not be considered as Wilms tumours. These include clear cell sarcoma and rhabdoid tumours (Fig. 14.1). Wilms tumour treatment, including an anthracycline, has been effective in clear cell sarcoma, but the results for the rhabdoid subtype have been disappointing. It is now generally accepted that the rhabdoid tumours should be treated much more intensively, particularly if there is spread beyond the renal capsule.

Molecular pathology

Although the WT1 gene has provided a fascinating paradigm for molecular carcinogenesis, the presence of mutation in tumour is not of any prognostic significance. Hyperploidy has been shown to be associated with unfavourable histology and poor outcome. More recently mutations affecting p53 have been described in a small percentage of tumours with poor outcome.

Staging

Role of CT scan in detecting lung metastases

Both commonly used staging systems (NWTS and SIOP) (Tables 14.1 and 14.2) are based on plain chest X-ray, including a PA and lateral films. This will underestimate the incidence of small lung metastases when compared with CT scanning. To what extent it is appropriate to upstage patients on the basis of lung CT alone remains unclear. Despite this, many study groups now base stage on this imaging modality. There is an argument that patients with small metastases, detectable only on lung CT scan, should be treated only with vincristine and actinomycin D so that information may be gathered regarding the significance of small

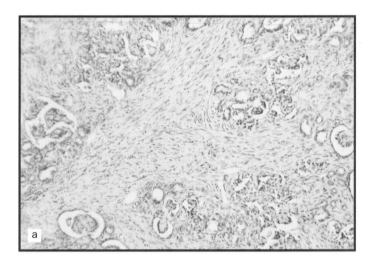
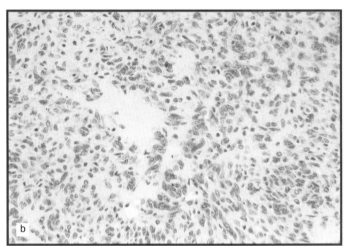
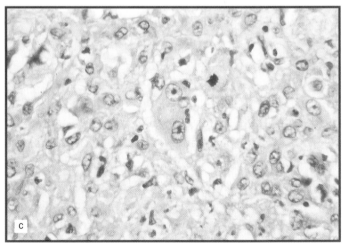

Figure 14.1 *Histological features of Wilms tumour. (a) Triphasic; (b) clear cell sarcoma; (c) rhabdoid.*

bulk deposits. The implications of upstaging from Stage I to Stage IV on treatment are significant, with regard to early morbidity, the need for central venous line insertion and potential cardiac and pulmonary toxicity. Moreover, in some protocols, alklylating agents are

Table 14.1 The NWTS staging system	
Stage	Characteristics
I	Tumour limited to the kidney and completely excised. Surface of renal capsule intact; no tumour rupture; no residual tumour apparent beyond margin of excision
II	Tumour extends beyond kidney but is completely excised; regional extension of tumour; vessel infiltration; tumour biopsy or local spillage of tumour confined to flank. No residual tumour apparent at or beyond margins of excision
III	Residual non-haematogenous tumour confined to the abdomen. Lymph node involvement of hilum, periaortic chains or beyond; diffuse peritoneal contamination by tumour spillage; peritoneal implants; tumour extends beyond resected margins, either microscopically or macroscopically; tumour not completely removable because of local infiltration into vital structures
IV	Deposits, beyond Stage III, in lung, liver, bone, brain
V	Bilateral renal involvement at diagnosis

used for this subgroup. In the event of relapse after two-drug therapy, the cure rate using multiagent chemotherapy and lung irradiation (i.e. similar standard Stage IV treatment) is likely to be high.

Detection of caval involvement

If a policy of primary surgery rather than preoperative chemotherapy is followed, caval involvement is the most important factor in determining inoperability (Fig. 14.2). Venocavagram through pedal veins is now rarely used and high-resolution Doppler ultrasound, CT scan or MRI are now the investigations of choice. MRI is probably the most sensitive and accurate method of distinguishing infiltration from external compression, although no imaging technique is completely infallible (Figs. 14.3 and 14.4).

Management

Surgery

The timing of surgery is largely determined by the study protocol with which the child is being treated. With the

Table 14.2 TNM grouping and staging system for Wilms tumour

(a) Grouping

Group	Characteristics
T: primary tumour	
TX	Primary tumour cannot be assessed
T0	No evidence of primary tumour
T1	Unilateral tumour 80 cm^2 or less in area (including kidney)
T2	Unilateral tumour more than 80 cm^2 in area (including kidney)
T3	Unilateral tumour rupture before treatment
T4	Bilateral tumours
N: regional lymph nodes	
NX	Regional lymph nodes cannot be assessed
N0	No regional lymph node metastasis
N1	Regional lymph node metastasis
M: distant metastasis	

(b) Staging

Stage	Primary tumour	Regional lymph nodes	Distant metastasis
I	T1	N0	M0
II	T2	N0	M0
III	T1	N1	M0
	T2	N1	M0
	T3	Any N	M0
IVA	T1	Any N	M1
	T2	Any N	M1
	T3	Any N	M1
IVB	T4	Any N	Any M

NWTS, virtually all patients with non-metastatic disease have attempted resection, including those with nodal involvement. Subsequent management is based on surgical staging, at which time histological subtype is defined. Conversely, with the SIOP strategy, no patient has primary surgery and no patient is biopsied. The diagnosis is based on clinical evidence and even

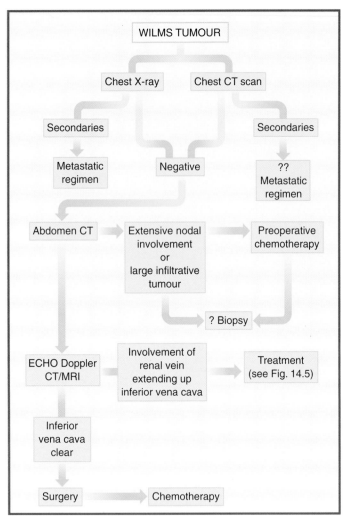

Figure 14.2 *Algorithm for treatment of Wilms tumour.*

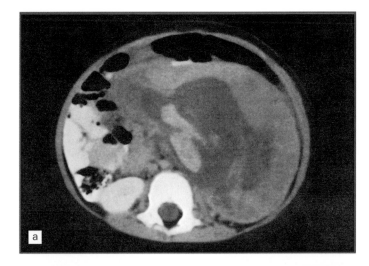

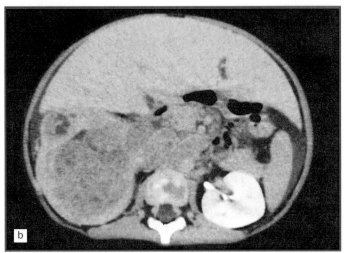

Figure 14.3 *Wilms tumour. (a) Typical CT scan showing large venous lakes; (b) CT scan showing extensive nodal infiltration.*

patients with small, easily resectable tumours receive vincristine and actinomycin D (VA). Outside formal trials, a more pragmatic approach may be followed, such as that shown in Figure 14.2. A decision whether to give preoperative chemotherapy is based on discussion with an experienced paediatric surgeon. If primary surgery is felt to be feasible, then most patients will end up being surgical Stage I and receive only VA. Patients with difficult tumours, including caval involvement, are given preoperative chemotherapy with VA ± doxorubicin (AVA) and, following delayed surgery, subsequent chemotherapy is based on the completeness of resection. A current UKCCSG randomised trial addresses the issue of preoperative chemotherapy versus surgery in operable tumours. It is hoped this will clarify the implications of downstaging patients with more extensive tumour by two-drug preoperative chemotherapy and, in particular, whether

this adversely affects the outcome of those patients who, in the past, would have received more intensive chemotherapy. Extensive caval involvement presents a particular challenge, requiring close collaboration between chemotherapists, radiologists and surgeons (Fig. 14.5). The only indication for surgery in this situation is if intracardiac tumour is causing significant dysfunction. Full cardiothoracic support is required, with appropriate bypass facilities.

Radiotherapy

In many national protocols, radiotherapy is given in all Stage II and III patients irrespective of preoperative chemotherapy. Whether radiotherapy is really necessary in the case of incomplete initial resection is controversial and is largely avoided by primary chemotherapy. Stage III tumour after delayed surgery is a more convincing indication for irradiation.

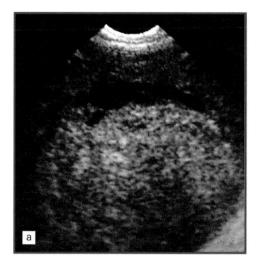

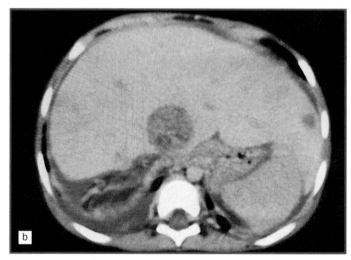

Figure 14.4 *Vena cava overlying large Wilms tumour. (a) Imaged using ultrasound; (b) CT scan demonstrating caval infiltration up the hepatic vein.*

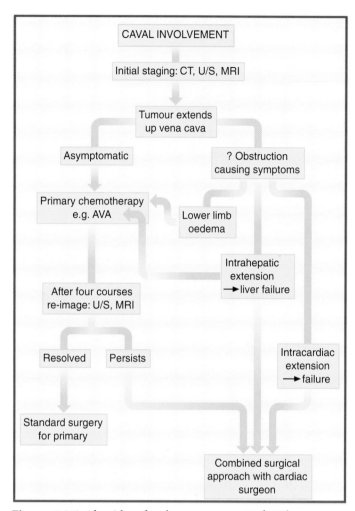

Figure 14.5 *Algorithm for the management of Wilms tumour with caval involvement.*

The role of radiation in lung metastases is also contentious. It is standard in the NWTS and UK but in the SIOP protocol if there is an adequate chemotherapy response radiation is omitted if at all possible. This reduces late sequelae with regard to thoracic cage growth and exacerbation of anthracycline-induced cardiomyopathy (Fig. 14.6).

Chemotherapy

A series of randomised trials run by NWTS have shown that short-duration actinomycin D and vincristine is adequate for Stage I patients and that more prolonged combination of actinomycin and vincristine and no irradiation is adequate for Stage II. In the SIOP 9 protocol, where patients are given preoperative chemotherapy, further chemotherapy is more aggressive after surgery if still Stage II and all receive

the addition of an anthracycline. Moreover, the Stage II node-positive patients also receive 15 Gy local radiotherapy. The NWTS 4 study further addresses the issue of treatment duration. Figure 14.7 outlines the strategy for the unusual bilateral (Stage V) tumours.

What approach should be used for unfavourable histology? For anaplastic tumours, NWTS Stage I lesions may be treated with the same chemotherapy approach as for favourable histology. For Stage II and beyond, more intensive chemotherapy, including cyclophosphamide and local irradiation, is recommended by the NWTS. For clear cell sarcoma, including Stage I, an intensive three- or four-drug regimen plus irradiation is advised. For rhabdoid tumours, there is still no satisfactory treatment; combination regimens including ifosfamide, etoposide and carboplatin are being evaluated.

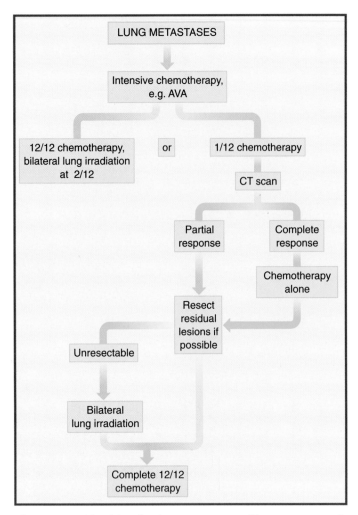

Figure 14.6 *Algorithm for the management of lung metastases in Wilms tumour.*

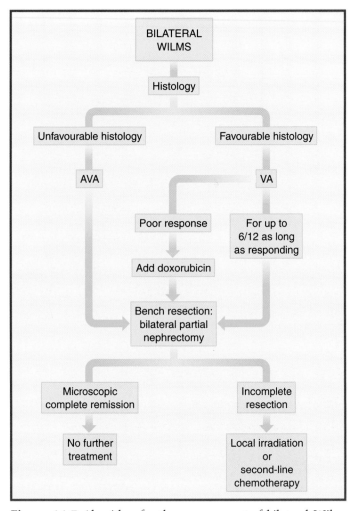

Figure 14.7 *Algorithm for the management of bilateral Wilms tumour.*

Management of metastatic sites other than lung

Liver tolerance at doses around 20 Gy may be poor and there is a high risk of radiation-enhanced veno-occlusive disease associated with vincristine and actinomycin D. Consumptive thrombocytopenia may be seen in the absence of overt veno-occlusive disease. Lesions in the brain or bone should also be treated with local irradiation following intensive primary chemotherapy; outcome is likely to be poor.

Management of recurrent disease

Although it is often believed that the overall cure rate for relapsed patients is relatively high, at least two publications have shown that only half of patients who are treated with vincristine or vincristine plus actinomycin D for Stage I disease and relapse can be cured with subsequent treatment. The outcome is bleaker for patients who receive three-drug therapy, renal bed irradiation or have unfavourable histology (Table 14.3). Consequently, more aggressive second-line chemotherapy regimens, including other active agents such as cyclophosphamide, etoposide and carboplatin have been devised (Figs. 14.8 and 14.9). The role of high-dose therapy with haematopoietic stem cell rescue remains unclear. Encouraging initial results have been reported using high-dose melphalan, either alone or in combination with carboplatin and etoposide. Follow-up is somewhat preliminary, but in high-risk patients it is logical to take advantage of the proven efficacy of high-dose melphalan in this tumour.

Table 14.3 Treatment and outcome in relapsed Wilms tumour after UKCCSG WT1 protocol

Stage of disease at presentation, initial histology and survival

Stage of disease	No. of patients	No. with favourable histology	Survival (No. of patients)	No. with unfavourable histology	Survival (No. of patients)
I	11	9	6	2	1
II	11	10	5	1	0
III	23	11	0	12	1
IV	21	16	3	5	0
V	5	5	1	–	0
Total	71	51	15	20	2

Treatment given after relapse

Treatment	No. of patients
Surgery	2
Radiotherapy	3
Chemotherapy	22
Surgery/chemotherapy	12
Surgery/radiotherapy	1
Chemotherapy/radiotherapy	18
Chemotherapy/radiotherapy/surgery	7
No treatment	6

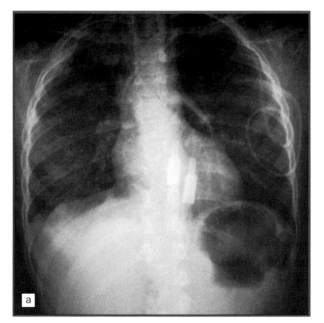 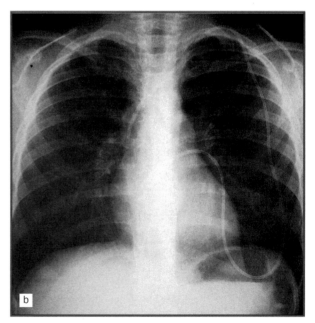

Figure 14.8 *Excellent response to second-line chemotherapy in relapsed metastatic Wilms tumour using cyclophosphamide, etoposide and carboplatin. (a) Pre-second-line treatment; (b) after treatment.*

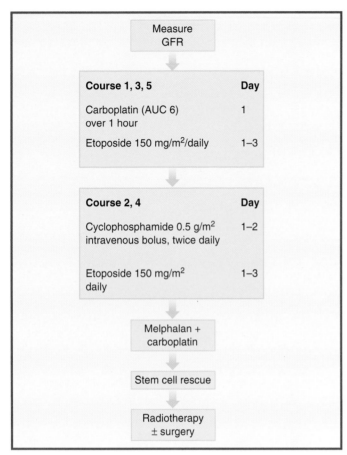

Figure 14.9 *Outline strategy for relapsed Wilms tumour previously treated with AVA ± radiotherapy.*

Further reading

Coppes, M.J., Zandvoort, S.W., Sparling, C.R. *et al.* (1992) Acquired von Willebrand disease in Wilms tumour patients. *Journal of Clinical Oncology* 10: 422–427.

D'Angio, G.J., Breslow, N., Beckwith, J.B. *et al.* (1989) The treatment of Wilms tumour. Results of the Third National Wilm's Tumour Study. *Cancer* 64: 349–360.

D'Angio, G.J., Evans, A.E., Breslow, N. *et al.* (1981) The treatment of Wilms tumour: results of the Second National Wilms Tumor Study. *Cancer* 47: 2302–2311.

de Camargo, G. and France, E.L. (1994) A randomised clinical trial of single dose versus fractionated dose dactinomycin in the treatment of Wilms tumour. *Cancer* 73: 3081–3086.

de Kraker, J., Lemerle, J., Voute, P.A. *et al.* (1990) Wilms tumour with pulmonary metastases at diagnosis: the significance of primary chemotherapy. *Journal of Clinical Oncology* 8: 1187–1190.

Garventa, A., Hartmann, O., Bernard, J.-L. *et al.* (1994) Autologous bone marrow transplantation for pediatric Wilms tumour: the experience of the European bone marrow transplantation solid tumour registry. *Medical and Pediatric Oncology* 22: 11–14.

Green, D.M., Fernbach, D.J., Norkool, P. *et al.* (1991) The treatment of Wilms tumor patients with pulmonary metastases detected only with computed tomography: a report from the National Wilms Tumor Study. *Journal of Clinical Oncology* 9: 1776–1781.

Green, D.M., Finklestein, J.Z., Norkool, P. *et al.* (1988) Severe hepatic toxicity after treatment with single-dose dactinomycin and vincristine. *Cancer* 62: 270–273.

Groot-Loonen, J.J., Pinkerton, C.R., Morris-Jones, P.H. and Pritchard, J. (1990) How curable is relapsed Wilms tumour? *Archives of Disease in Childhood* 65: 968-970.

Grundy, P., Breslow, N., Green, D.M. *et al.* (1989) Prognostic factors for children with recurrent Wilms tumour: results from the second and third National Wilms Tumour Study. *Journal of Clinical Oncology* 7: 638–647.

Lemerle, J., Voute, P.A., Tournade, M.F. *et al.* (1983) Effectiveness of preoperative chemotherapy in Wilms tumour: results of an International Society of Pediatric Oncology (SIOP) clinical trial. *Journal of Clinical Oncology* 1: 604–609.

Pinkerton, C.R., Groot-Loonen, J.J., Morris-Jones, P.H. and Pritchard, J. (1991) Response rates in relapsed Wilms tumor. *Cancer* 67: 567–571.

Pritchard, J., Imeson, J., Barnes, J. *et al.* (1995) Results of the United Kingdom Children's Cancer Study Group (UKCCSG) first Wilms tumor study (UKW1). *Journal of Clinical Oncology* 13: 124–133.

Sorensen, K., Levitt, G., Sebag-Montefiore, D. *et al.* (1995) Cardiac function in Wilms tumour survivors. *Journal of Clinical Oncology* 13: 1546–1556.

CHAPTER 15
Rhabdomyosarcoma

C.R. Pinkerton

Introduction

Considerable progress has been made regarding the molecular basis and use of molecular pathology in rhabdomyosarcoma, both for diagnosis and prognosis. Because of the widely varying sites of disease and the broad age range of those affected, planning therapy represents a particular challenge to the paediatric oncologist. Unlike many other tumours, there is a need for considerable individualisation of treatment strategies. Primary chemotherapy followed by surgery, and in some cases local radiotherapy, is often the treatment of choice, but this approach will vary depending on the site, age, pathological subtype and initial response to treatment.

Clinical prognostic variables

Staging systems

Over the last few years there has been some convergence of the differing approaches to the initial staging of soft tissue sarcoma in children. The European groups (SIOP) have applied the TNM classification, which separates those with nodal involvement or loco-regional extension from those with localised disease (Tables 15.1 and 15.2). The Intergroup Rhabdomyosarcoma Study (IRS) has emphasised the importance of postsurgical staging, irrespective of the extent of initial disease on imaging (Table 15.3). Analysis of IRS data has shown that the former approach is probably more appropriate and this has led to the increased trend towards primary chemotherapy, getting away from the problems

associated with often disfiguring or mutilating radical primary surgery.

In comparing the results of the SIOP and IRS groups, it is important to take note of the different staging systems and, in the past, the differing attitude to primary chemotherapy. As will be discussed below, there are some subgroups where even SIOP investigators have reservations about depending entirely on primary chemotherapy. In the future, there may be a move back to the use of radiotherapy to improve local control rates. In previous studies, node involvement has emerged as one of the most important adverse prognostic factors and, as has been the case in the IRS, any distant metastatic site reduces the likelihood of disease-free survival.

Pathological subgroups

The most common subgroups of rhabdomyosarcoma are illustrated in Figure 15.1. Those with botryoid tumours do well, but this may reflect favourable sites and likelihood of complete resectability. The spindle cell variant, which often is associated with para-testicular or non-parameningeal head and neck tumours, also appears to be particularly favourable, but again this may reflect the tumour site. There is no doubt that those with the alveolar subgroup do less well, but this to some extent reflects the unfavourable sites and age of the patient. Controversy has surrounded the precise definition of alveolar rhabdomyosarcoma, with much debate regarding the significance of small components in an otherwise embryonal tumour and also how to distinguish the solid alveolar variant. Recent collaborative work between the IRS and SIOP histopathologists has

Table 15.1 Presurgical TNM staging for rhabdomyosarcoma	
Group	Characteristics
T: primary tumour	
TX	The minimum requirements to assess the primary tumour cannot be met
T0	No evidence of primary tumour
T1	Tumour confined to the organ or tissue of origin
T1a	Tumour 5 cm or less in its greatest dimension
T1b	Tumour more than 5 cm in its greatest dimension
T2	Tumours involving one or more contiguous organs or tissues or with adjacent malignant effusion, or multiple tumours in the same organ (more than one tumour is considered as a primary tumour with distant metastases)
T2a	Tumour 5 cm or less in its greatest dimension
T2b	Tumour more than 5 cm in its greatest dimension
N: regional lymph nodes	
NX	The minimum requirements to assess the regional lymph nodes cannot be met; in cases where the regional lymph nodes cannot be assessed clinically or radiologically, NX should be considered as N0 in stage I and II
N0	No evidence of regional lymph node involvement
N1	Evidence of regional lymph node involvement
M: distant metastases	
MX	The minimum requirements to assess the presence of distant metastases cannot be met
M0	No evidence of distant metastases
M1	Evidence of distant metastases

Table 15.2 Postsurgical histopathological classification of rhabdomyosarcoma	
Group	Characteristics
pT: primary tumour	
pTX	The extent of local invasion cannot be assessed
pT0	No evidence of tumour found on histological examination of specimen
pT1	Tumour limited to organ or tissue of origin; excision complete and margins histologically free
pT2	Tumour with invasion beyond the organ or tissue of origin; excision complete and margins histologically free
pT3	Tumour with or without invasion beyond the organ or tissue of origin; excision incomplete
pT3a	Evidence of microscopic residual tumour
pT3b	Evidence of macroscopic residual tumour on biopsy only
pT3c	Adjacent malignant effusion regardless of the size
pN: regional lymph nodes	
pNX	The extent of invasion cannot be assessed No pathological examination of the lymph nodes performed or inadequate information on the pathological findings
pN0	No evidence of tumour found on histological examination of regional lymph nodes
pN1	Evidence of invasion of regional lymph nodes
pN1a	Evidence of invasion of regional lymph nodes; involved nodes considered to be completely resected
pN1b	Evidence of invasion of regional lymph nodes; involved nodes considered to be incompletely resected

attempted to reach a consensus regarding this matter – any alveolar component is now deemed significant. Currently, on the SIOP and IRS regimens more intensive treatment is given to those with alveolar histology. Because of the difficulties mentioned above, it is important that rapid central review is available to confirm this decision is appropriate.

Role of molecular pathology

The almost invariable association of the t(2;13) or t(1;13) translocation with alveolar histology has led to this being used to support the diagnosis (Figure 15.2). FISH or RT–PCR methodology is used to detect the transcript. To what extent these translocations are found in non-alveolar tumour remains to be determined in large prospective studies. Loss of heterozygosity on chromosome 11 may provide supportive evidence of the embryonal subtype, but this has not been clearly addressed in a large study. The adverse impact of diploidy or tetraploidy remains contentious, with differing results from various groups. Although the IRS suggest this should be used to stratify patients, this has not been the view of the SIOP to date. Similarly, the striking adverse

Table 15.3 IRS clinical group system for staging rhabdomyosarcoma

Clinical group		Extent of disease and surgical result
I	A	Localised tumour, confined to site of origin, completely resected
	B	Localised tumour, infiltrating beyond site of origin, completely resected
II	A	Localised tumour, gross total resection, but with microscopic residual disease
	B	Locally 'extensive' tumour (spread to regional lymph nodes), completely resected
	C	'Extensive' tumour (spread to regional lymph nodes), gross total resection but with microscopic residual disease
III	A	Localised or locally extensive tumour, gross residual disease after biopsy only
	B	Localised or locally extensive tumour, gross residual disease after 'major' resection (≥50% debulking)
IV		Any size primary tumour, with or without regional lymph node involvement, with distant metastases, irrespective of surgical approach to primary tumour

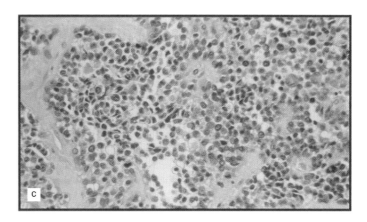

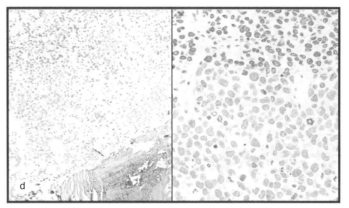

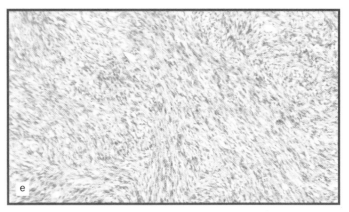

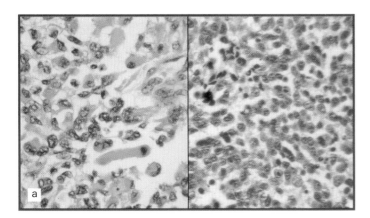

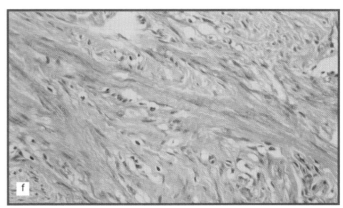

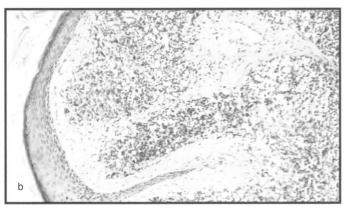

Figure 15.1 *Histological features of rhabdomyosarcoma. (a) Typical embryonal; (b) botryoid; (c, d) alveolar; (e) fibrosarcoma; (f) fibromatosis.*

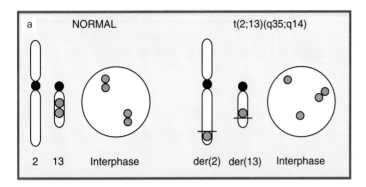

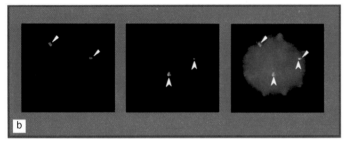

Figure 15.2 *FISH demonstration of t(2;13) translocation. As shown in both the schema (a) and interphase (b) preparations, the different colour probes that flank the site of translocation are separated in tumour cells carrying t(2;13).*

prognostic impact claimed to be associated with the expression of the MDR-1 gene or P-glycoprotein has not been confirmed by subsequent studies.

Staging methodology

Clear definition of loco-regional extension and involvement of local nodes are probably the most important factors in staging these tumours. The use of lymphangiography or node dissection in paratesticular disease may detect minimal involvement, but these are of little value with regard to ultimate outcome and have been replaced by high-resolution CT scanning. The decision whether to use MRI or CT scan will depend on the site of tumour. Because of movement artifact, MRI of the abdomen may be inferior to CT scanning, whereas delineation of soft tissue masses at other sites is better with MRI. Bony erosion appears to be of prognostic significance in parameningeal tumours and, therefore, a combination of MRI and CT may be appropriate at this site. The incidence of bone or bone marrow disease in patients with localised node-negative primaries is negligible and investigations for these are, therefore, unnecessary. As in the case of other small round cell tumours, bilateral bone marrow aspirate and trephine are required in patients with more advanced primary tumours. There

is interest in the use of RT–PCR to demonstrate the t(2;13) or t(1;13) transcript in bone marrow in these patients, which may ultimately prove to be of prognostic significance. Bone scan should be limited to those with loco-regional extension or nodal involvement.

The risk groupings based on site and pathology currently used by the SIOP group are shown in Tables 15.4 and 15.5. This is contrasted with the risk groups used in IRS IV (Table 15.6).

Management

Treatment issues at different sites
Orbit

Although a comparatively rare site, management of orbital tumour is one of the most contentious issues. Very high cure rates are achieved with simple chemotherapy, such as vincristine and actinomycin D, associated with localised irradiation. In the younger child, such local irradiation may be associated with significant cosmetic sequelae, both in terms of orbital bone growth and cataracts. In the older child with small primary tumours and using high-quality radiotherapy, these sequelae should be minimal. The alternative approach followed by the SIOP group is the use of primary chemotherapy, restricting local irradiation to where there is evidence on imaging of

Table 15.4 The SIOP risk groupings of sites	
Site	Comment
Orbit	Without involvement of parameningeal sites or local bone destruction
Head and neck	Non-parameningeal sites
Head and neck	Parameningeal sites[a] (including orbit or other site with extension to a parameningeal site)
Genitourinary tract	Bladder, prostate
Genitourinary tract	Paratestis, vagina, uterus
Limbs	
Other sites	
[a] Parameningeal sites: head and neck, nasopharynx, nasal cavity, paranasal sinus, middle ear/mastoid, pterygoid fossa; orbit with intracranial tumour or with bone destruction; paraspinal tumours with intraspinal, extradural extension.	

Site	TNM stage[a]				
	IpT1	IpT2 and pT3a, b, c	II	III	IV
Orbit: NPM	–	3	3	3	4
Head and neck: NPM	1	3	3	3	4
Head and neck, orbit: PM	–	–	3	3	4
Genitourinary tract					
Bladder, prostate	1	3	3	3	4
Vagina, uterus, paratestis	1	2	2	3	4
Limbs	1	3	3	3	4
Other	1	3	3	3	4

Table 15.5 Risk groupings for MMT 95

NPM, non-parameningeal sites; PM, parameningeal sites
[a] Risk groupings: 1, low risk; 2, standard risk; 3, high-risk non-metastatic; 4, metastatic. All non-metastatic alveolar tumours are allocated to the high-risk group regardless of site or stage.

residual tumour that is not amenable to complete surgical resection. Unfortunately the last approach has been associated with a worryingly high local failure rate. This has led to the use of increasingly intensive primary chemotherapy, which invariably carries with it both early and late morbidity. It seems likely that, in

the future, treatment at this site will be stratified with regard to tumour size and the age of the child. Vincristine, actinomycin (VA) plus local irradiation is probably the treatment of choice for the older child, where high-precision local radiotherapy may be used. In contrast, the small child with the bulky primary tumour in whom more extensive radiation will be mandatory, a primary chemotherapy approach, accepting the potential sequelae of chemotherapy, is preferable (Figs. 15.3a, b).

Middle ear

Middle ear tumours are usually of botryoid subtype and, therefore, are highly chemosensitive. The middle ear is a particularly difficult site at which to confirm a complete remission with imaging. Surgical confirmation of complete remission may risk sacrificing hearing on that side. In this setting, it may be appropriate to have a low threshold for the use of consolidation radiotherapy, particularly in the older child. This should not adversely affect hearing but will guarantee local control.

Parameningeal sites

The parameningeal sites are one area where there is no argument regarding the necessity for elective local

Table 15.6 Risk grouping system adapted for IRS IV

Stage	Sites	Tumour invasiveness[a]	Tumour size[a]	Node stage[a]	Metastatic stage[a]
1	Orbit	T1 or T2	a or b	N0 N1 or NX	M0
	Head and neck				
	Genitourinary				
2	Bladder, prostate	T1 or T2	a	N0 or NX	M0
	Extremity				
	Cranial parameningeal				
	Other				
3	Bladder, prostate	T1 or T2	a	N1	M0
	Extremity	T1 or T2	b	N0 N1 or NX	M0
	Cranial parameningeal				
	Other				
4	All	T1 or T2	a or b	N0 or N1	M1

[a,b] See Table 15.1.

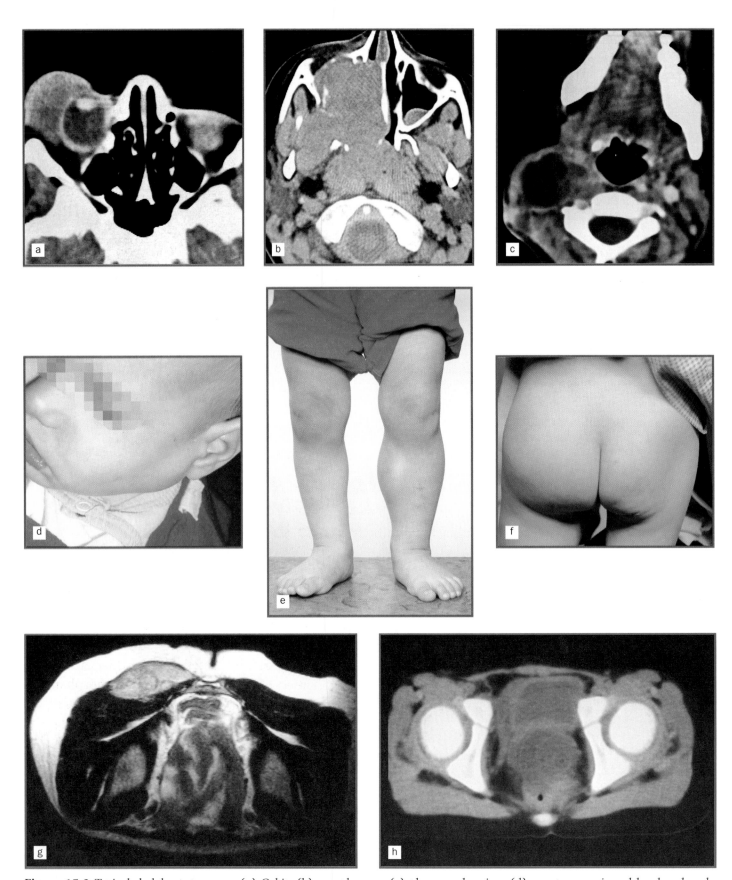

Figure 15.3 *Typical rhabdomyosarcoma. (a) Orbit; (b) nasopharynx; (c) pharyngeal region; (d) non-parameningeal head and neck; (e) limb; (f, g) buttock; (h) pelvis.*

irradiation. The definition of parameningeal sites is given in Table 15.4. The policy of the IRS is to deliver radiotherapy concurrently with initial chemotherapy during the first few weeks. This may be associated with severe toxicity, particularly mucositis, but appears to have highest local control rate. A significant improvement in outcome for this subgroup has been seen in IRS III, but this may reflect more accurate planning of radiotherapy. The role of intrathecal treatment is unproved and this has been dropped from both the SIOP and current IRS protocols, unless there is evidence of CSF infiltration. In this situation, the combination of intrathecal cytosine and methotrexate is used, although unproved. These are not the most active drugs in rhabdomyosarcoma but the choice of chemotherapy is limited by route. Paraspinal tumours are not generally regarded as falling within this subgroup, and even if there is intraspinal extension, provided the tumour proves chemosensitive, a similar approach may be followed to that at other sites.

Non-parameningeal head and neck sites
The head and neck is a favourable site and consequently there is the possibility of avoiding late effects of chemotherapy by primary surgery to achieve complete removal of a non-parameningeal primary tumour (Fig. 15.3c, d). This decision requires considerable discussion with head and neck plastic surgeons, as in the younger child one would have major reservations about the long-term cosmetic sequelae of radical surgery. However, with smaller tumours, it is probably appropriate to attempt a complete removal, as this avoids the risk of cyclophosphamide-induced sterilisation, which could be regarded of more importance in later life than some facial scarring. As in the case of orbital tumours, this is a classic example of the dilemma facing the paediatric oncologist when trying to weigh up the relative importance of different late sequelae in patients who are likely to be cured of their tumour.

Limb
Rhabdomyosarcoma of the limb are often of alveolar subtype and, therefore, require aggressive adjuvant chemotherapy, such as ifosfamide, vincristine,

actinomycin (IVA), even if there has been complete resection of the primary tumour (Fig. 15.3e). The role of local radiotherapy is unproved and if there has been complete removal of the primary tumour this is probably not necessary. More aggressive surgery is justified at this site because of the poorer outcome, particularly if local control is not achieved. There is, however, no place for debilitating surgery, and amputation is no longer considered in first-line treatment.

Intra-abdominal tumours
Intra-abdominal tumours almost invariably require intensive chemotherapy as primary treatment approach (Fig. 15.3f–h). There may be associated ascites, although the prognostic significance of positive cytology is unclear. The same applies to the rare intrathoracic tumour where a pleural effusion contains tumour cells. Although by current definitions these tumours are not regarded as metastatic, it seems likely that they will do at least as poorly as those with nodal involvement and, therefore, a more intensive chemotherapy approach is appropriate. In the current SIOP protocol this would involve a six-drug regimen.

Bladder/prostate
Although the SIOP approach of attempting to conserve a functioning bladder by using primary chemotherapy has been adapted by the IRS group, there remain reservations about this strategy. Longer-term follow-up has shown that a significant percentage ultimately require cystectomy or have received local radiotherapy because of failure to achieve complete remission. The consequence is a poor functioning bladder caused by a combination of radiotherapy and cyclophosphamide-induced cystitis. Despite this, all patients should be given the option of attempting to conserve the bladder and surgery restricted to removal of postchemotherapy residual mass (Figs. 15.3h and 15.4).

Where conservative surgery has been applied and apparent complete remission achieved using chemotherapy, there is the issue of follow-up using cystoscopy. Repeat biopsies of bladder may be difficult to interpret and there are an increasing number of anecdotal reports of apparent rhabdomyoblastic infiltration on follow-up cystoscopic biopsies that have not progressed, and also children who have had

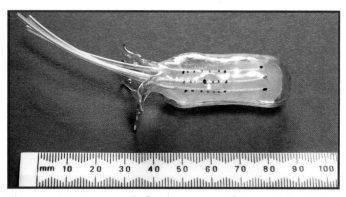

Figure 15.4 *A cast made for the purpose of interstitial radiation for a vaginal rhabdomyosarcoma.*

cystectomies because of positive cystoscopic biopsies in whom no active tumour was found in the resected specimen. One should, therefore, be wary about acting on the outcome of such biopsies and central review of specimens is advisable before any radical action is taken.

Paratesticular tumours

How intensive chemotherapy must be in the case of a completely resected paratesticular tumour remains unclear. In an attempt to avoid sterilisation, a conservative approach has been used by the SIOP group, using a short course of vincristine and actinomycin D. This necessitates accurate initial staging. Lymphadenectomy or lymphangiography are no longer used but it is important to guarantee complete microscopic clearance at the level of the spermatic cord and node negativity using high-resolution CT or MRI. If these are in doubt, more

intensive chemotherapy should be given as salvage may be difficult in the event of nodal recurrence.

Management of metastatic disease

Recent analysis carried out by both IRS and SIOP groups has shown that the outcome of these patients can be predicted on the basis of age and site of metastases. Those over 10 years of age with bone or bone marrow disease are virtually incurable, whereas the younger child with lung metastases alone may have up to a 40% chance of cure.

What type of chemotherapy should be used? The strategy in both SIOP and IRS is a multiagent regimen incorporating all of the active agents currently available for this tumour type. Consolidation of complete remission with high-dose melphalan has been evaluated by SIOP in a sequential study of six-drug versus six-drug plus melphalan regimens. This has, however, failed to show any significant improvement in overall survival. There have been a number of single-arm studies, both in Europe and the USA, using a range of combinations, but data from the European Bone Marrow Transplant Registry have shown little evidence of any benefit from single or multiagent chemotherapy or from TBI-based combinations. The UKCCSG has recently piloted a high-dose combination regimen involving pulsed cyclophosphamide, etoposide and carboplatin with peripheral blood stem cell (PBSC) rescue (Fig.

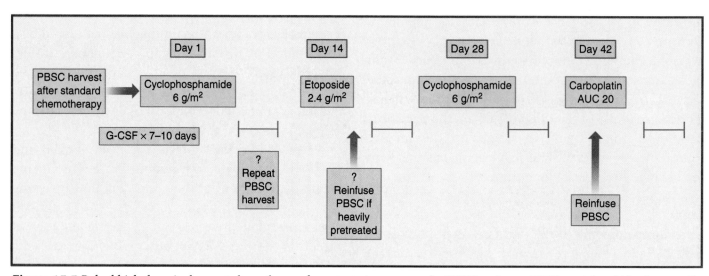

Figure 15.5 *Pulsed high-dose single agent chemotherapy for metastatic sarcoma: the CECC regimen. PBSC, peripheral blood stem cells.*

15.5). It is planned to introduce this early in treatment, followed by a continuing chemotherapy phase for up to 12 months.

The role of lung irradiation remains unclear. This has been a standard part of the IRS strategy and may account for the apparently better outcome in those with lung metastases. This has been omitted from recent SIOP studies but will be reincorporated in the new trial. As with other sarcomas, the issue of whether a total dose of up to 18 Gy to the lungs is really likely to add any significant anti-tumour effect in this aggressive subtype remains debatable. Similarly, it seems illogical to irradiate sites of bone abnormalities, which almost certainly reflect only a small percentage of tumour foci.

What should be the timing of stem cell harvest prior to high-dose therapy? As these patients may present with bone marrow involvement, it is unwise to attempt PBSC harvest until there is clear evidence of complete marrow remission. As in neuroblastoma, it is possible that growth factor-primed PBSC harvesting may mobilise tumour cells from bone marrow. Ongoing studies using RT–PCR to detect minimal levels of tumour transcript address this issue and may throw light on the optimal timing. In patients with no overt bone or bone marrow disease, harvest can probably occur after one or two courses. This would apply to approximately half the patients, in whom pulsed high-dose chemotherapy with PBSC rescue could be incorporated as early as possible in treatment.

Management of relapsed tumours

Figure 15.6 outlines an approach for the management of relapsed tumours. Therapy will depend on the initial extent of disease and intensity of chemotherapy. It should be emphasised that there is no role for high-dose therapy in patients whose disease is progressing on second- or third-line chemotherapy, except in the setting of phase II trials. EBMT data have shown no benefit in this subgroup and indeed little to any other group except perhaps those with local nodal relapse. As a general principle, it seems inappropriate to use chemotherapy agents to which the patient has been previously exposed; therefore, if the relapse occurs within 6 months of treatment or on treatment then different drugs should, if possible, be used in second-line therapy. Alternative scheduling such as oral etoposide or rapid delivery etoposide/cisplatin has

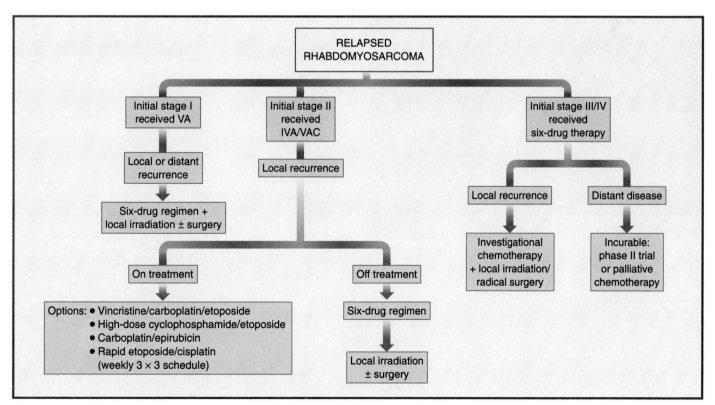

Figure 15.6 *Algorithm for the management of relapsed rhabdomyosarcoma.*

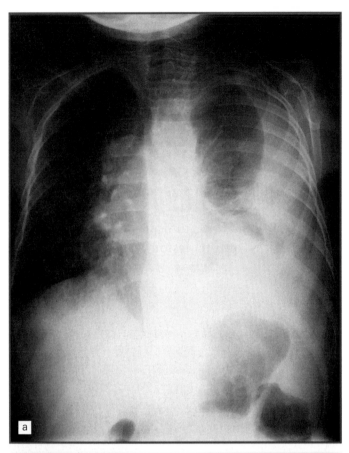

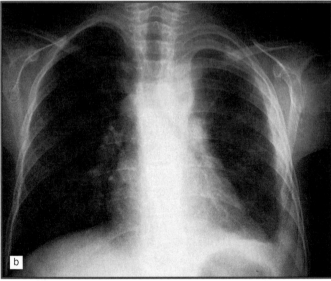

Figure 15.7 *Recurrent rhabdomyosarcoma following an intensive six-drug regimen and high-dose chemotherapy showing a dramatic response to simple 21-day oral etoposide. (a) Pre-treatment; (b) post-treatment with etoposide.*

been evaluated (Fig. 15.7; Box 15.1). A more liberal attitude to the use of extended-field radiotherapy and radical surgery is necessary if cure is to be achieved.

Box 15.1 Palliative chemotherapy

Oral etoposide for 21 days
Low-dose doxorubicin weekly
Doxorubicin continuous infusion
Oral etoposide, 3 × per week × 21 days
Oral cyclophosphamide, daily

Novel treatments

There is considerable interest in the value of topoisomerase I inhibitors, such as topotecan (camptothecin) and irinotecan (CPT11). Xenograft data both from the St Jude and the Villejuif group have shown these to be highly active. CPT11 is currently going to phase II trial in the UK and France and topotecan is under evaluation in the USA.

The high percentage of tumours overexpressing P-glycoprotein, particularly at relapse, have raised the possibility of MDR modulation in this tumour type. High-dose cyclosporin has been incorporated in first-line treatment of high-risk patients, but in the absence of control groups these data will be difficult to interpret. Novel agents such as PSC 833 are entering phase II evaluation and ultimately should be incorporated in a randomised phase III study.

Management of non-rhabdomyoma soft tissue sarcoma

Clinical data regarding the chemosensitivity of tumours such as synovial sarcoma, fibrosarcoma, malignant fibrous histiocytoma (Fig. 15.8) or undifferentiated liposarcoma are limited. In general, if these tumours are small then radical surgery alone is probably sufficient. There is some controversy regarding the role of adjuvant chemotherapy in this situation, but unlike in rhabdomyosarcoma there is no proven benefit. Where tumours are unresectable (Fig 15.9), it is appropriate to give two or three courses of IVA to evaluate chemosensitivity, as response rates as high as 40% have been described.

Fibromatosis or desmoid tumours may present a particular problem. Low-dose chemotherapy with vincristine and actinomycin D may be effective in fibromatosis, although responses are likely to be slow.

Curability will depend on the ability to achieve complete resection following chemotherapy (Fig. 15.10).

Management of infantile fibrosarcoma can be difficult, as the natural history of these tumours remains unclear. In general, a relatively conservative approach is appropriate and in some cases spontaneous stabilisation of growth or even involution may occur. Of particular difficulty, may be differentiation between infantile fibrosarcoma, fibromatosis and haemangiopericytoma, as there can be considerable overlap with regard to pathological features and it may be difficult to predict the likely aggressiveness of the lesion (Fig. 15.10). Where chemotherapy is indicated, it may be appropriate to

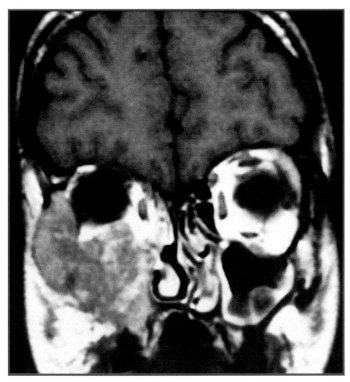

Figure 15.8 *Malignant fibrohistiocytoma arising in a patient treated four years previously for an orbit rhabdomyosarcoma. This proved to be chemo- and radio-resistant.*

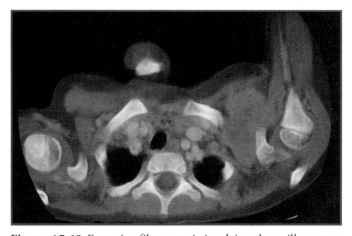

Figure 15.10 *Extensive fibromatosis involving the axillary area. This was chemo-resistant and surgically unresectable.*

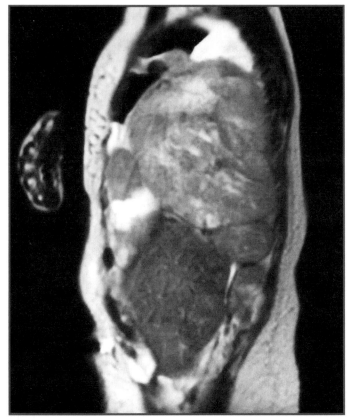

Figure 15.9 *Very extensive fibrosarcoma affecting the upper abdomen. This was totally chemoresistant and clearly unresectable.*

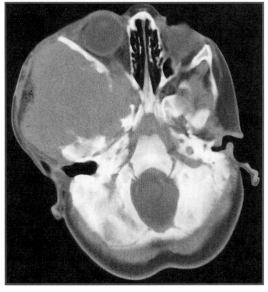

Figure 15.11 *Fibrosarcoma in a 18-month-old infant. This failed to respond to IVAD and local radiotherapy but a partial response was achieved with weekly vincristine, actinomycin and 21-day oral etoposide.*

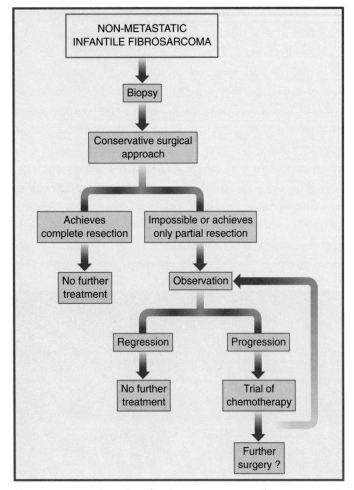

Figure 15.12 *Algorithm for the management of non-metastatic infantile fibrosarcoma. Chemotherapy with vincristine and actinomycin D is recommended as first-line treatment given every three weeks.*

start with a relatively simple vincristine/actinomycin-based regimen, proceeding to a more intensive multiagent protocol in the event of a poor response (Figs. 15.11 and 15.12).

Further reading

Asmar, L., Gehan, E.M., Newton, W.A. Jr et al. (1994) Agreement among and within groups of pathologists in the classification of rhabdomyosarcoma and related childhood sarcomas: report of an international study of four pathology classifications. *Cancer* 74: 2579–2588.

Birch, J.M., Hartely, A.L., Blair, V. et al. (1990) Cancer in the families of children with soft tissue sarcoma. *Cancer* 66: 2239–2248.

Carli, M., Morgan, M., Bisogno, G. et al. (1995b) Malignant peripheral nerve sheath tumours in childhood (MPNST). A combined experience of the Italian and German co-operative studies. SIOP XXVII Meeting. *Medical and Pediatric Oncology* 25: 243.

Carli, M., Perilongo, G., Cordero di Montezemolo, L. et al. (1987) Phase II trial of cisplatin and etoposide in children with advanced soft tissue sarcoma: a report from the Italian Co-operative Rhabdomyosarcoma Group. *Cancer Treatment Reports* 71: 525–527.

Carli, M., Pinkerton, R., Frascella, E. et al. (1995a) Metastatic soft-tissue sarcomas in children: preliminary results of the second European Intergroup Study (EIS) MMT-91. *Medical and Pediatric Oncology* 25: 256.

Cavazzana, A.O., Schmidt, D., Ninfo, V. et al. (1992) Spindle cell rhabdomyosarcoma: a prognostically favorable variant of rhabdomyosarcoma. *American Journal of Pathology* 16: 229–235.

Chan, H.S., Thorner, P.S., Haddad, G. and Ling, V. (1990) Immunohistochemical detection of P glycoprotein: prognostic correlation in soft tissue sarcoma of childhood. *Journal of Clinical Oncology* 8: 689–704.

Crist, W.M., Garnsey, L., Beltangady, M. et al. (1990) Prognosis in children with rhabdomyosarcoma: a report of the Intergroup Rhabdomyosarcoma Studies I and II. *Journal of Clinical Oncology* 8: 443–452.

Crist, W., Geham, E.A., Ragab, A.H. et al. (1995) The third Intergroup Rhabdomyosarcoma Study. *Journal of Clinical Oncology* 13: 610–630.

Frascella, E., Pritchard-Jones, K., Modak, S. et al. (1996) Response of previously untreated metastatic rhabdomyosarcoma to combination chemotherapy with carboplatin, epirubicin and vincristine. *European Journal of Cancer* 32A: 821–825.

Heyn, R., Ragab, A., Romey, B. et al. (1986) Late effects of therapy in orbital rhabdomyosarcoma in children. A report from the Intergroup Rhabdomyosarcoma Study. *Cancer* 57: 1738–1743.

Horowitz, M.E., Kinsella, T.J., Wexler, L.H. et al. (1993) Total-body irradiation and autologous bone marrow transplant in the treatment of high-risk Ewing's sarcoma and rhabdomyosarcoma. *Journal of Clinical Oncology* 11: 1911–1918.

Horowitz, M.E., Pratt, C.B., Webber, L. et al. (1986) Therapy for childhood soft-tissue sarcomas other than rhabdomyosarcoma: a review of 62 cases. *Journal of Clinical Oncology* 4: 559–564.

Koscielniak, E., Jurgens, H., Winkler, K. et al. (1993) Treatment of soft tissue sarcoma in childhood and adolescence. *Cancer* 70: 2557–2567.

Koscielniak, E., Rodary, C., Flamant, F. et al. (1992) Metastatic rhabdomyosarcoma and histologically similar tumors in childhood. A retrospective European multicenter analysis. *Medical and Pediatric Oncology* 20: 209–215.

Maurer, H.M., Gehan, E.A., Beltangady, M. et al. (1993) The Intergroup Rhabdomyosarcoma Study–II. *Cancer* 71: 1904–1922.

Miser, J.S., Kinsella, T.J., Triche, T.J. et al. (1987a) Ifosfamide with mesna uroprotection and etoposide: an effective regimen in the treatment of recurrent sarcomas and other tumors of children and young adults. *Journal of Clinical Oncology* 5: 191–198.

Niggli, F.K., Powell, J.E., Parkes, S.E. et al. (1994) DNA ploidy and proliferative activity (S-phase) in childhood soft-tissue sarcomas: their value as prognostic indicators. *British Journal of Cancer* 69:1106–1110.

Ninane, J. (1991) Chemotherapy for infantile fibrosarcoma. *Medical and Pediatric Oncology* 19: 209.

Olive, D., Flamant, F., Zucker, J.M. et al. (1984) Paraaortic lymphadenectomy is not necessary in the treatment of localized paratesticular rhabdomyosarcoma. *Cancer* 54: 1283–1287.

Otten, J., Flamant, F., Rodary, C. et al. (1989) Treatment of rhabdomyosarcoma and other malignant mesenchymal tumors of childhood with ifosfamide + vincristine + dactinomycin (IVA) as front-line therapy. *Cancer Chemotherapy and Pharmacology* 24 (Suppl.): 30.

Pappo, A.S., Shapiro, D.N., Crist, W. and Maurer, H.M. (1995)

Biology and therapy of pediatric rhabdomyosarcoma. *Journal of Clinical Oncology* 13: 2123–2139.

Pinkerton, C.R., Groot-Loonen, J., Barrett, A. *et al.* (1991) Rapid VAC, high dose melphalan regimen. A novel chemotherapy approach in childhood soft tissue sarcomas. *British Journal of Cancer* 64: 381–385.

Raney, B., Tefft, M., Newton, W.A. *et al.* (1987) Improved prognosis with intensive treatment of children with cranial soft tissue sarcomas arising in nonorbital parameningeal sites. *Cancer* 59: 147–155.

Regine, W.F., Fontanesi, J., Kumar, P. *et al.* (1995) A phase II trial evaluating selective use of altered radiation dose and fractionation in patients with unresectable rhabdomyosarcoma. *International Journal of Radiation Oncology, Biology and Physics* 31: 779–805.

Rodary, C., Gehan, E., Flamant, F. *et al.* (1991) Prognostic factors in 951 nonmetastatic rhabdomyosarcoma in children: a report from the International Rhabdomyosarcoma Workshop. *Medical and Pediatric Oncology* 19: 89–95.

Rousseau, P., Flamant, F., Quintana, E. *et al.* (1994) Primary chemotherapy in rhabdomyosarcomas and other malignant mesenchymal tumors of the orbit: results of the International Society of Pediatric Oncology MMT 84 study. *Journal of Clinical Oncology* 2: 516–521.

Soule, E.H. and Pritchard, D.J. (1977) Fibrosarcoma in infants and children. A review of 110 cases. *Cancer* 40: 1711–1721.

Weiss, A.J. and Lackman, R.D. (1989) Low-dose chemotherapy of desmoid tumours. *Cancer* 64: 1192–1194.

CHAPTER 16

Hepatoblastoma and hepatocellular carcinoma

C.R. Pinkerton

Introduction

Primary liver tumours in childhood account for around 5% of childhood neoplasms and over two-thirds occur within the first year of life (Figs. 16.1–16.3). Metastatic deposits in liver most commonly occur with soft tissue sarcoma and Wilms tumour (Fig. 16.4). Diffuse or focal infiltration may be evident in neuroblastoma (Fig. 16.5). The biology and behaviour of hepatoblastoma (HBL) and hepatocellular carcinoma (HCC) differ but the therapeutic strategy is similar for both tumours.

A number of biological clues have recently emerged regarding the character of hepatoblastoma, with the demonstration of loss of heterozygosity on chromosome 11p15 in a number of tumours and also the association between hepatoblastoma and familial polyposis coli. The FAP gene has been located in chromosome 5q. These observations are a further justification for initial biopsy to obtain suitable tissue for studying the molecular basis of this tumour.

Diagnosis

In over 80% of HBL and in over 60% of HCC raised levels of alpha-fetoprotein (AFP) are detected. As with germ cell tumours this is useful both for diagnosis and response assessment. Rate of AFP decline correlates with outcome. It could be argued that with the presence of a liver mass and raised AFP no further investigations are required, as the chemotherapy is the same for HBL and HCC. This approach will, however,

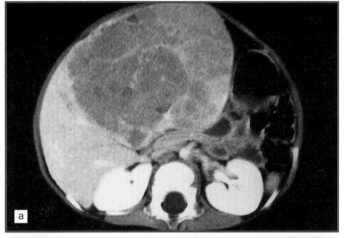

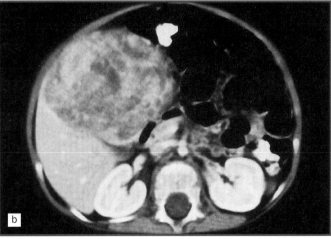

Figure 16.1 *Hepatoblastoma. (a) CT scan before four courses of PLADO (cisplatin/doxorubicin) chemotherapy; (b) CT scan after chemotherapy.*

lead to misdiagnosis of the rare intrahepatic teratoma. Moreover, as a significant percentage of masses following chemotherapy are found to be entirely necrotic, a firm diagnosis may not be achieved at the time of postchemotherapy resection. There is now a

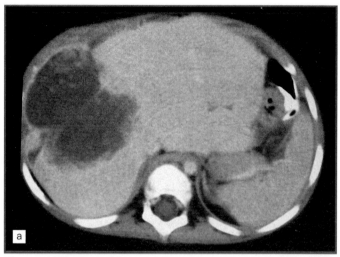
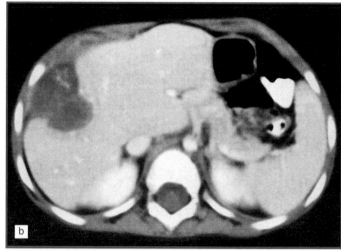

Figure 16.2 *Hepatoblastoma showing significant shrinkage following four courses of PLADO chemotherapy.*

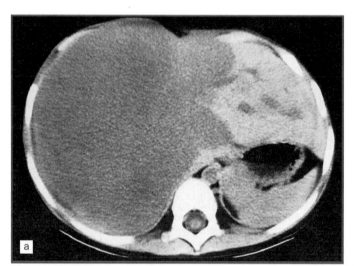
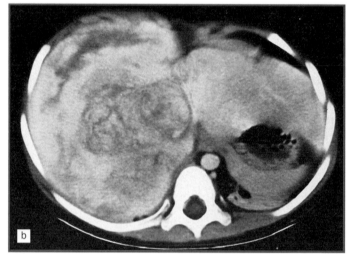

Figure 16.3 *Massive intrahepatic sarcoma. (a) CT scan; (b) MR imaging.*

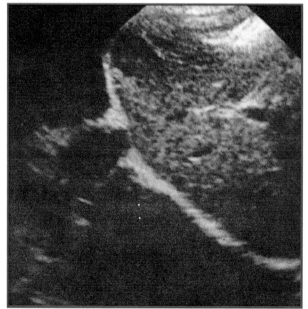

Figure 16.4 *Hepatic metastasis in Wilms tumour shown on ultrasound.*

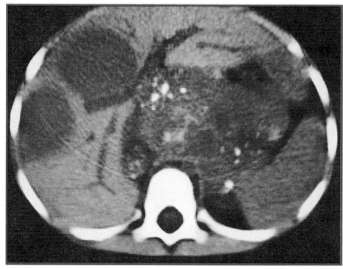

Figure 16.5 *Intrahepatic metastases associated with abdominal neuroblastoma.*

general consensus that provided there is no significant risk associated with biopsy this should be done. In the case of a very unwell infant with massive hepatic disease, or an associated coagulopathy, a biopsy may be contraindicated on clinical grounds.

The differential diagnoses of an isolated hepatic mass in the child are listed in Table 16.1 and the tumours summarised in Table 16.2.

Table 16.1 Differential diagnoses for an isolated hepatic mass	
Benign causes	Malignant causes
Developmental cysts	Hepatoblastoma
Mixed hamartoma	Hepatocelluar carcinoma
Focal nodular hyperplasia	
Hepatocellular adenoma	
Nodular regenerative hyperplasia	
Haemangioendothelioma	Embryonal sarcoma
Cavernous haemangioma	Angiosarcoma
Mesenchymal hamartoma	Rhabdomyosarcoma
Inflammatory pseudotumour	Rhabdoid tumour
Teratoma	Yolk sac tumour

Table 16.2 Relative incidence of hepatic tumours	
Tumour type	Proportion of hepatic tumours (%)
Hepatoblastoma	28–43
Hepatocellular carcinoma	15–23
Haemangioendothelioma	13–27
Embryonal sarcoma	6–8
Mesenchymal hamartoma	6
Focal nodular hyperplasia	2–7
Adenoma	2–5

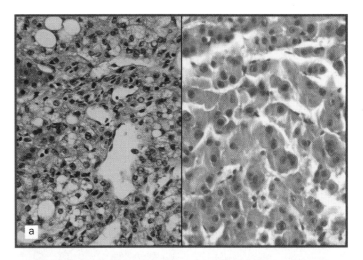

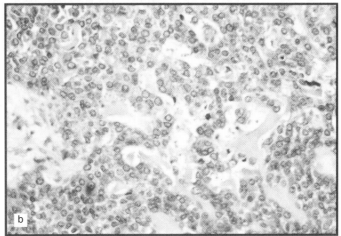

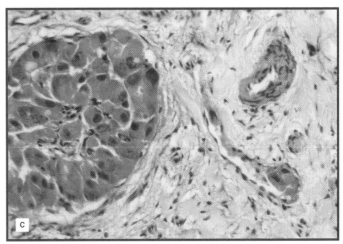

Figure 16.6 *Histological variants of primary hepatic tumours. (a) Fetal hepatoblastoma; (b) embryonal hepatoblastoma: (c) fibrolamellar hepatocellular carcinoma.*

Pathological variants

Hepatoblastoma can be classified into a range of subgroups, although the prognostic significance of these are unclear (Fig. 16.6). Seventy-five per cent are epithelial, subdivided into fetal and embryonal types and the remainder are mixed epithelial or mesenchymal. An anaplastic variant of the last has been defined, and this morphologically poorly differentiated tumour may have a worse outcome. Conversely, patients with pure fetal histology, particularly those with small localised tumours, may do better. At the present time, however, no stratification is made on the basis of pathology. The fibrolamellar variant of HCC is associated with a lower degree of chemosensitivity. If complete resection is achieved, it has a favourable outlook but in the presence of non-localised and unresectable disease the outcome is particularly poor.

Staging

Hepatic tumours are generally divided into localised and metastatic disease. The majority of distant metastases are in the lung, although bone may be involved. Of more importance is the staging of the primary tumour (Fig. 16.7). Even with effective primary chemotherapy, surgery has a vital role to play in achieving cure (Fig. 16.8). Few patients are long-term survivors if complete resection is not achieved. The SIOP pretreatment grouping system is shown in Figure 16.7.

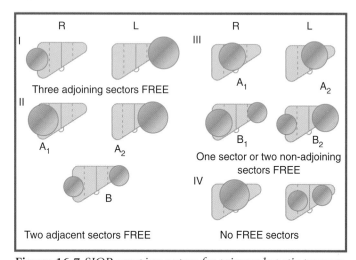

Figure 16.7 *SIOP grouping system for primary hepatic tumours.*

Management

Is surgery alone ever adequate for HBL and HCC? This is unlikely, but how minimal chemotherapy can be remains to be defined. The current SIOP study is evaluating the role of single-agent cisplatin in both resected and small volume primary disease. It has been previously demonstrated that single-agent doxorubicin

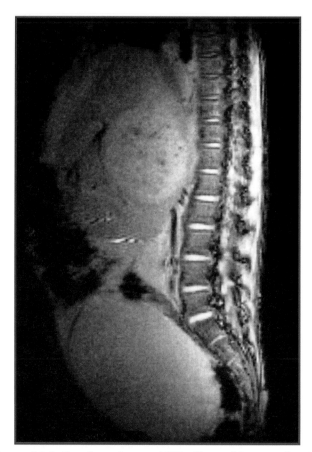

Figure 16.8 *Postchemotherapy MRI of hepatoblastoma showing well-circumscribed lesion amenable to surgical resection. Complete clearance was achieved.*

is adequate to eliminate undetected micrometastatic disease. Because of the efficacy of primary chemotherapy in HBL, primary resection is generally restricted to small group I tumours.

What chemotherapy should be used? The relatively simple PLADO regimen appears to be as effective as any other combination regimen. Although there was initial concern about late effects with regard to cardiac toxicity and impaired renal function, the introduction of a continuous infusion regimen for both cisplatin and doxorubicin has significantly reduced these toxicities. More complex regimens incorporating 5-fluorouracil, vincristine and ifosfamide appear to add little compared with the PLADO regimen (Box 16.1).

Management of relapsed disease

Phase II studies in adults with HCC and limited data in children with HBL have shown ifosfamide to be an active agent. Etoposide has also been used in HCC but

Box 16.1 Chemotherapy regimens in hepatoblastoma

PLADO: cisplatin, doxorubicin

Cisplatin, doxorubicin, ifosfamide

Cisplatin, vincristine, 5-fluorouracil

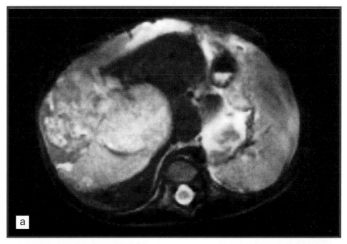

results are somewhat less encouraging. Figure 16.9 outlines a proposed strategy for patients with relapsed disease. Primary refractory disease may respond to similar second-line regimens but outcome is generally poor (Fig. 16.10).

When should liver transplantation be considered?

Liver transplantation is usually limited to children with unresectable but chemosensitive primary tumours, either HBL or HCC, where more than one lobe is involved, i.e. group III or group IV. Transplantation may be the only way of achieving complete remission. If this is judged to be likely on

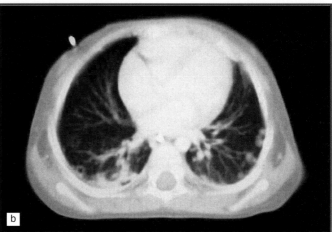

Figure 16.10 (a, b) *Hepatoblastoma imaged with MRI: despite some shrinkage of the primary site, there was little change in the lung metastases, thus precluding definitive surgery.*

initial imaging, discussions should be held at an early stage with transplant surgeons to ensure that the child is put on the waiting list for urgent transplantation.

The issue in children with lung metastases is less clear. For HBL, where the cure rate now exceeds 70% for such patients, provided the tumour is chemosensitive but the primary remains unresectable there is justification for transplantation. The difficulty is to persuade the transplant surgeon that the child is of sufficiently high priority to compete with other needy cases. There is often discussion about how long one should wait to demonstrate that the chemotherapy has been effective. In this 'Catch 22' situation, waiting to provide sustained complete remission of lung metastases may result in progression of the residual intrahepatic disease; it is, therefore, advisable to seek a co-operative surgeon who is prepared to perform transplant immediately at the end of standard chemotherapy, provided lung metastases have cleared.

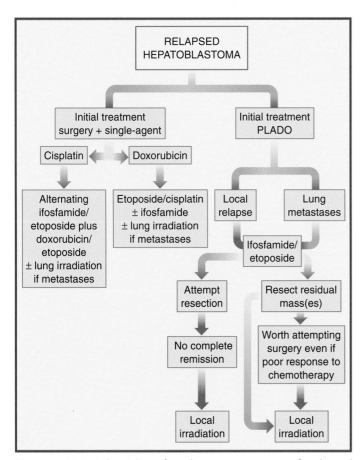

Figure 16.9 *Algorithm for the management of relapsed hepatoblastoma.*

Is there a role for surgery to lung metastases? HBL, along with osteosarcoma and Wilms tumour, is one of the tumours in which lung metastases may be genuinely localised and, therefore, surgical exploration of postchemotherapy residual imageable lesions is justified. There have even been reports of long-term remission following resection of chemoinsensitive lung metastases in HBL, and with a limited number of deposits this should be considered.

What is the role of local radiotherapy? Lung irradiation is not necessary in chemosensitive lung metastases in HBL, although in the older child with HCC this could be considered. Beneficial effect of local irradiation to sites of microscopic residual disease following incomplete postchemotherapy resection remains controversial, but in the absence of any other option and the knowledge that microscopic disease at this stage invariably progresses, there is an argument for its use. Obviously the dose and field must be limited and sophisticated planning by experienced paediatric radiotherapists is mandatory.

Further reading

Black, C.T., Luck, S.R., Musemeche, C.A. *et al.* (1991) Aggressive excision of pulmonary metastases is warranted in the management of childhood hepatic tumours. *Journal of Pediatric Surgery* 26: 1082–1985.

Conran, R.H., Hitchcock, C.L., Waclawiw, M.A. *et al.* (1992) Hepatoblastoma: the prognostic significance of histologic type. *Pediatric Pathology* 12: 167–183.

Douglass, E.C., Reynolds, M., Finegold, M. *et al.* (1993) Cisplatin, vincristine, and fluorouracil therapy for hepatoblastoma: a Pediatric Oncology Group Study. *Journal of Clinical Oncology* 11: 96–99.

Habrand, J.L., Nehme, D., Kalifa, C. *et al.* (1992) Is there a place for radiation therapy in the management of hepatoblastoma and hepatocellular carcinomas in children? *International Journal of Radiation Oncology, Biology and Physics* 23: 675–676.

Koneru, B., Flye, M.W., Busuttil, W. *et al.* (1991) Liver transplantation for hepatoblastoma: the American experience. *Annals in Surgery* 213: 118–121.

MacKinlay, G.A. and Pritchard, J. (1992) A common language for childhood liver tumours. *Pediatric Surgery International* 7: 325–326.

Ninane, J., Perilongo, G., Stalens, J.P. *et al.* (1991) Effectiveness and toxicity of cisplatin and doxorubicin (PLADO) in childhood hepatoblastoma and hepatocellular carcinoma: a SIOP pilot study. *Medical Pediatric Oncology* 19: 199–203.

Ortega, J.A., Douglass, E., Feusner, J. *et al.* (1994) A randomized trial of cisplatin (DDP)/vincristine (VCR)/ 5-fluorouracil (5FU) vs DDP/doxorubicin (DOX) in continuous infusion for the treatment of hepatoblastoma. Results from the Pediatric Intergroup Study (CCG-8881/POG-8945). ASCO Abstracts *Journal of Clinical Oncology* 13: 416.

Shafford, E.A. and Pritchard, J. (1993) Extreme thrombocytosis as a diagnostic clue to hepatoblastoma. *Archives of Disease in Childhood* 68: 88–90.

Stringer, M.D., Henayake, S., Howard, E.R. *et al.* (1995) Improved outcome for children with hepatoblastoma. *British Journal of Surgery* 82: 386–391.

van Tornout, J.M., Buckley, J.D., Quin, J.J. *et al.* (1997) Timing and magnitude of decline in alpha-fetoprotein levels in treated children with unresectable or metastatic hepatoblastoma are predictors of outcome: a report from the Children's Cancer Group. *Journal of Clinical Oncology* 15: 1190–1197.

von Schweinitz, D., Wischmeyer, P., Leuschner, I. *et al.* (1994) Clinico-pathological criteria with prognostic relevance in hepatoblastoma. *European Journal of Cancer* 30: 1052–1058.

CHAPTER 17

Malignant germ cell tumours

C.R. Pinkerton

Introduction

The three most common sites of malignant germ cell tumour (MGCT) are the sacrococcyx, occurring in the neonate and young infant, the ovary, often occurring in the early teens, and the testis, occurring either in the infant or adolescent (Table 17.1).

Four pathological subtypes of MGCT predominate in childhood, namely yolk sac tumour, chorio-carcinoma, germinoma and embryonal carcinoma. The features of each of these are typical (Fig. 17.1) but a mixed pattern is frequently seen.

Does histological subtype influence outcome?

Although in adults very high levels of AFP and pure yolk sac histology may be a poor prognostic factor, this is not the case in childhood. There is no evidence that any of the main histological subtypes are any less chemosensitive to modern cisplatin-based regimens than another. The one histological subtype where there remains some controversy is the immature teratoma. The features of this subtype are shown in Figure 17.1c. Immature teratomas most commonly occur in the ovary, where they may make up to 10% of tumours. This usually involves children in their early teens. Although it has been suggested that adjuvant chemotherapy is necessary in such tumours, which are usually completely resected, this has little basis. The situation has been confused because of inclusion of patients with mixed tumours, as indicated by raised AFP or human β-chorionic gonadotrophin (β-HCG)

levels. Although in adults, metastases have been reported with immature teratoma, this does not appear to be the case in childhood. The mainstay of treatment is, therefore, surgical, and following incomplete resection a 'wait and watch' policy is justified. Elective use of chemotherapy is not indicated. In the event of tumour recurrence, there is little evidence that the ultimate cure rate is compromised by such a conservative policy.

Are molecular genetics of diagnostic or prognostic value?

In adult testicular tumours, aneuploidy and iso-chromosome 12p are common findings. It has been suggested that the latter may be present in virtually all testicular tumours, if sensitive detection methods such as FISH are used. The abnormality appears to be present irrespective of the pathological subtype, being found in embryonal carcinoma, seminoma and yolk sac tumour, and indicates its possible role in pathogenesis. In paediatric practice, isochromosome 12p is generally only found in adolescent testicular or mediastinal disease. In children under 5 years of age, where yolk sac tumour predominates, isochromosome 12p is generally not found. Tumours are normally diploid or tetraploid. Loss of chromosome 1, particularly deletion of 1p36, chromosome 3 and 6 have been reported. None of these cytogenetic abnormalities are of prognostic significance, but their detection in residual tumour following chemotherapy may be of relevance with regard to the malignant potential of the residual mass. It is also of

Table 17.1. Relative incidence of malignant germ cell tumours according to age and pathology

Site	Relative incidence	Age	Pathology
Sacrococcyx	35	Neonate	Teratoma Mature 65%, immature 5%
			Malignant 10–30%
Ovary	25	Early teens	Teratoma
			Mature 65%, immature 5%
			Malignant 30% (pure yolk sac 30%, mixed 30%)
Testis	20	Infant and adolescent	Teratoma Mature 20%, malignant 80% (yolk sac 90%, germinoma 10%)
			Embryonal carcinoma 1–5%
Cranium	5	Child	Germinoma 20–50%
			Embryonal carcinoma 20–50%
			Mature teratomas 20–30%
Mediastinum	5	Adolescent	Teratoma
			Mature 60%, mixed 20%
			Embryonal carcinoma 20%
Retroperitoneum	5	Infant	Teratoma
			Mature or immature
			Rarely malignant
Head and neck	3	Infant and neonate	Usually mature teratoma
			Immature rarely malignant
Vagina	2	Infant	Usually yolk sac

note that haematological malignancies associated with germ cell tumours may exhibit isochromosome 12p. Such leukaemias have been blamed on the use of etoposide. The occurrence of isochrome 12p suggests that the leukaemia has arisen from the teratomatous population, rather than bone marrow, thus arguing against it being a consequence of topoisomerase II inhibition by etoposide. The gene for mast cell growth factor (MGF) is located at 12q22, which may explain the documented increased incidence of haematopoietic malignancies in association with, in particular, mediastinal germ tumour.

What staging systems should be used?

MGCT are one of the paediatric tumours in which there is the most urgent need for a restructuring of staging systems. These have been derived from adult classifications and have generally been site orientated (Tables 17.2 and 17.3) and, therefore, have used a separate system for ovarian, testicular and extragonadal tumours. With the advent of highly effective chemotherapy, these are now inappropriate. The aim of any staging system should be to distinguish patient groups on the basis of outcome, which is no longer the case with the older staging systems. Table 17.4 outlines an alternative system that may be more relevant to clinical practice in paediatrics. Moreover, it is applicable irrespective of tumour site. If treatment is to be further refined, limiting the very intensive regimens to high-risk patients, and omitting using agents with late effects in low-risk patients, it is critical that accurate and relevant staging systems are devised. This requires further collaboration between international

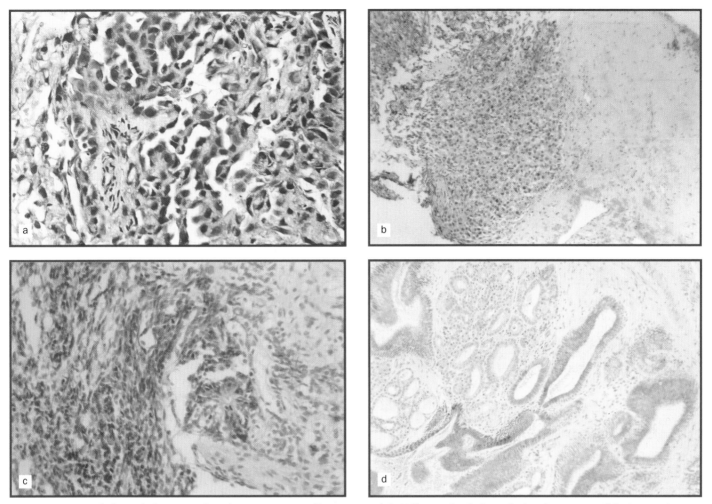

Figure 17.1 *Pathological features of malignant germ cell tumours. (a) Yolk sac (endodermal sinus) tumour; (b) dysgerminoma; (c) immature teratoma; (d) mature teratoma.*

Stage	Extent of disease
I	Limited to ovary or ovaries; peritoneal washings negative for malignant cells
	No clinical, radiographical or histological evidence of disease beyond the ovaries
	Tumour markers normal after appropriate postsurgical half-life decline
	The presence of gliomatosis peritonei does not up-stage patient
II	Microscopic residual or positive lymph nodes (≤2 cm as measured by pathologist)
	Peritoneal washings negative for malignant cells
	Tumour markers positive or negative
	The presence of gliomatosis peritonei does up-stage patient
III	Lymph node with malignant metastatic nodule (≤2 cm as measured by pathologist)
	Gross residual or biopsy only
	Contiguous visceral involvement (omentum, intestine, bladder)
	Peritoneal washings positive for malignant cells
	Tumour markers positive or negative
IV	Distant metastases, including liver

Table 17.2 POG/CCG staging of ovarian germ cell tumours

Table 17.3 POG/CCG staging of testicular tumours

Stage	Extent of disease
I	Limited to testes
	Completely resected by high inguinal orchidectomy or trans-scrotal orchidectomy with no spill
	No clinical, radiographical or histological evidence of disease beyond the testes
	Tumour markers normal after appropriate postsurgical half-life decline; patients with normal or unknown markers at diagnosis must have a negative ipsilateral retroperitoneal node dissection to confirm stage I
II	Trans-scrotal orchidectomy with gross spill of tumour
	Microscopic disease in scrotum or high in spermatic cord (≤5 cm from proximal end)
	Retroperitoneal lymph node involvement (≤2 cm)
	Increased tumour markers after appropriate half-life
III	Retroperitoneal lymph node involvement (≤2 cm)
	No visceral or extra-abdominal involvement
IV	Distant metastases, including liver

Table 17.4 Staging system for malignant germ cell tumours in childhood for all extracranial sites: ovary, testis and other extragonadal sites

Stage	Extent of disease
I	Complete resection of primary tumour with subsequent fall of markers
	No nodal involvement on CT or at surgery
II	Microscopic residual disease at surgical margins
	Trans-scrotal resection or biopsy
III	Gross residual disease or biopsy only ± nodes positive on imaging
	Contiguous visceral involvement in the case of ovary, i.e. omentum, intestine, bladder
	Diffuse tumour spill at surgery
IV	Distant metastases to liver, lung, bone, bone marrow, distant nodes, brain

groups to pool patient data and determine how best to stratify patients.

Who are currently the high-risk patients? In adults with disseminated disease, a number of adverse prognostic factors have been identified. These include the level of serum marker, bulk disease, sites and number of metastases. In paediatric patients, the initial level of marker is of less relevance than the decline and eventual return to normal. As in many other childhood tumours, the initial tumour bulk is likely to be an adverse factor. For example, massive mediastinal or large malignant sacrococcygeal tumours with extensive intra-abdominal distention may be more difficult to cure. Whether this is related to the difficulty in achieving complete surgical resection of any residual tumour after primary chemotherapy or to the initial tumour volume is difficult to determine. Bone or bone marrow are rare sites of metastasis in childhood but are probably also of adverse prognostic significance.

Surgical issues

Initial procedure

It is important that no surgery beyond a biopsy is performed until the staging results are to hand, as extensive surgery to the primary tumour is inappropriate if distant metastases are detected.

If the tumour is localised, the first decision is whether it is operable. Figures 17.2 and 17.3 illustrate large tumours in mediastinum and sacrococcyx, where although surgery may be technically feasible, because of potential early and late sequelae it is inappropriate.

The child with massive mediastinal disease and raised tumour markers

In all paediatric cancers, a biopsy is desirable, not only to confirm the diagnosis but also to document histological subtype and molecular biology. In the case of massive mediastinal disease, there may be significant potential respiratory embarrassment. Intubation for general anaesthesia can be hazardous and laryngeal or tracheal oedema following intubation for a biopsy procedure may result in the necessity for post-biopsy ventilation. This may compromise the commencement of appropriate chemotherapy. As in the case of mediastinal disease from other causes (e.g. T-cell lymphoma), a decision regarding biopsy requires careful clinical judgement. There may be situations where there is no supportive diagnostic evidence from serum AFP or HCG and one is left with a differential diagnosis of mediastinal teratoma, T-cell lymphoma or

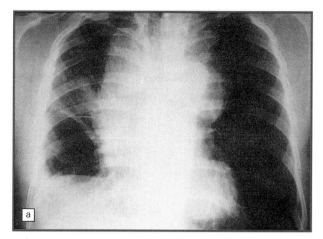

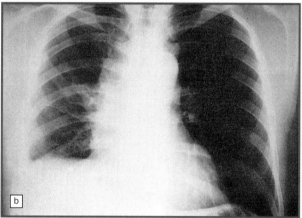

Figure 17.2 *Extensive mediastinal dysgerminoma associated with elevated HCG levels (a), showing excellent response to PVB chemotherapy (b).*

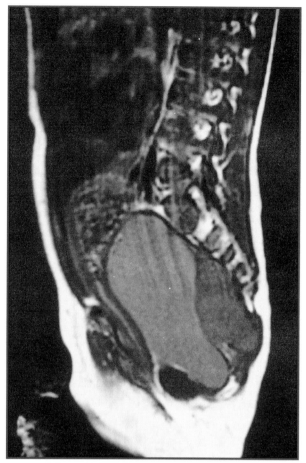

Figure 17.3 *Extensive sacrococcygeal teratoma presenting in a 6-month-old child. The extent of intrapelvic component is generally an adverse prognostic factor. This tumour recurred despite first- and second-line chemotherapy.*

Hodgkin's lymphoma. In this situation, empirical commencement of chemotherapy with vincristine and prednisolone may be appropriate. This may be sufficient to produce some cytoreduction that will facilitate a biopsy within 24–48 hours, following which appropriate chemotherapy may be commenced. Where markers are raised, immediate treatment with PVB or JEB may be started.

Ovarian tumours

Ovarian tumours are probably the site at which inappropriate surgery is most commonly performed. Occasionally, with marker-negative tumours and features characteristic of mature teratoma on CT scan, local resection is appropriate as the first procedure (Fig 17.4). With more advanced disease, there is no indication for aggressive primary surgery involving oophorectomy or salpingectomy. Surprisingly, these are still performed, with disastrous results on subsequent fertility. Often this

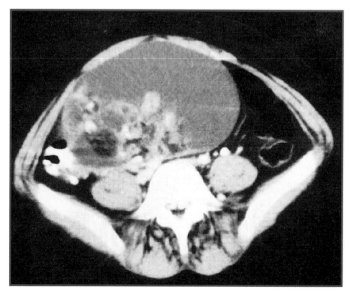

Figure 17.4 *Mature teratoma of right ovary on CT scan. This was associated with negative markers and was completely resected.*

is a result of a child presenting with an acute abdomen and at laparotomy extensive ovarian or pelvic disease is detected. The surgeon then feels committed to attempting resection, which is entirely inappropriate. In this situation, a biopsy alone should be taken and even if subsequent CT scanning shows that the tumour was potentially resectable, it is more appropriate to go back and do a second procedure that can be carefully planned from detailed imaging. More frequently, primary chemotherapy is commenced with conservative surgery at a later date.

Which patients may be cured with surgery alone?

In general, a wait-and-watch policy can be applied to MGCT at all sites if there is evidence of complete microscopic resection. The majority of patients will have an elevated serum marker at diagnosis (i.e. AFP or HCG), which can be estimated weekly to ensure the normal decline. Where there is no increased serum marker, careful ultrasound or CT follow-up is appropriate. In the event of local recurrence, cure rates are very high because of the exquisite chemosensitivity of these tumours.

Serum marker monitoring

Serum markers are useful, not only to document complete excision in localised tumour but also to follow response to primary chemotherapy. Although with chemotherapy, the decline in marker is somewhat less rapid than after surgical resection, this should still follow the normal elimination half-life. A slow decline indicates a degree of chemoresistance and will predict for a poor outcome.

It is essential that markers are followed for at least 18 months after cessation of treatment, as although tumour generally recurs within 12 months, it may occur for up to 2 years.

Serum marker that does not change after primary chemotherapy

What should be done if the serum marker shows little change after primary chemotherapy but imaging shows a reduction in tumour size? This indicates some degree of chemoresistance. In general, if the marker level returns to

normal after surgery, one would simply follow the patient's progress. There is no necessity to introduce second-line chemotherapy or local radiotherapy. However, if imaging suggests that complete resection is unlikely, or surgery is attempted and is incomplete, then a change to second-line chemotherapy is justified. If surgery is incomplete but the resected tumour is predominantly differentiated, then one should wait and see if markers fall to normal postoperatively. If so, no change in chemotherapy is required (Figs. 17.5 and 17.6).

How to react to rises in marker level off treatment?

The normal AFP level of 5 and HCG level of 10 IU/ml may be exceeded periodically during the 2-year follow-

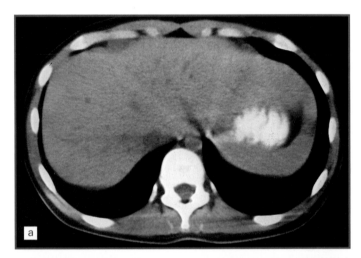

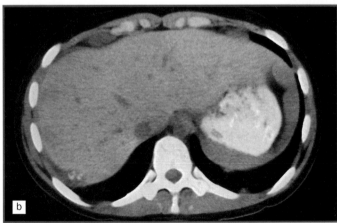

Figure 17.5 *CT scan showing metastases on surface of the liver of a girl with an ovarian germ cell tumour that showed mixed histological features associated with raised AFP (a). AFP returned to normal on BEP chemotherapy, but despite this, the metastases appeared to increase in size (b). No further chemotherapy was given but surgical exploration resulted in removal of multiple lesions that all were differentiated to teratoma. There was no recurrence of local disease.*

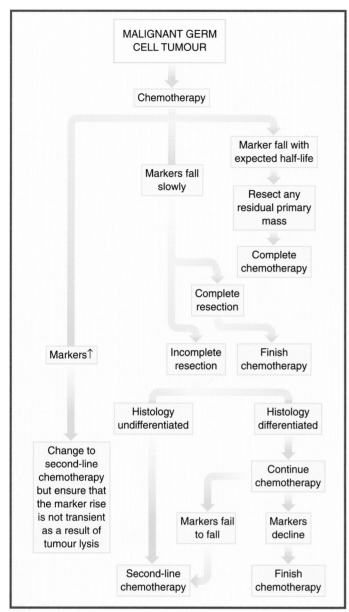

Figure 17.6 *Algorithm for marker interpretation in management of MGCT.*

up but this is rarely more than two or three times the normal baseline. Provided this is the case, no action is required. Potential causes of marker elevation may be liver trauma or hepatitis. Often there is no apparent cause. There should always be a high index of suspicion in the event of a rise in tumour marker and levels should be repeated weekly, rather than monthly, following an unexplained elevation. A useful general policy is to refrain from acting precipitously in the face of a rising serum marker. There is nothing to be lost by waiting and watching until the level is in three figures, and there can, therefore, be little doubt about the recurrence. At this point, extensive imaging is justified

to determine the site(s) of relapse. This should include CT or MRI of the original primary site, chest CT scan and bone scan. Although AFP scans have been used, they are not in current use. A difficult situation arises where the site of recurrent disease cannot be detected. In general, if the only evidence of recurrent disease was a high AFP, waiting is still appropriate and the site of recurrent disease will usually declare itself in due course (Figure 17.7).

Chemotherapy options

What chemotherapy to use? Table 17.5 outlines the range of chemotherapies that have been used in paediatric

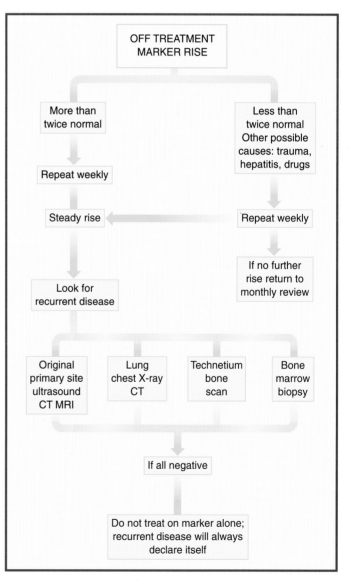

Figure 17.7 *Algorithm for approach to raised marker levels off treatment.*

Table 17.5 Chemotherapy regimens for paediatric germ cell tumours

Regimen	Components	Administration	
		Intravenous dose	Schedule
PVB	Cisplatin	20 mg/m²	Days 1–5
	Vinblastine	0.2 mg/kg	Days 1 and 2
	Bleomycin	15 units/m²	Days 2, 9, 16
BEP	Cisplatin	100 mg/m²	Day 1
	Etoposide	120 mg/m²	Days 1–3
	Bleomycin	15 units/m²	Day 2
JEB	Carboplatin	600 mg/m²	Day 1
	Etoposide	120 mg/m²	Days 1–3
	Bleomycin	15 units/m²	Day 2

practice. Currently, the gold standard is BEP, which is as effective as the original PVB regimen but better tolerated. The role of carboplatin remains controversial. UKCCSG data indicate that it is at least as effective as cisplatin, provided the dose is adequate. The dose is calculated on a formula based on kidney function (Box 17.1). Using an AUC of 6, which is somewhat higher than that generally used in adults, and accepting the consequent myelosuppression, the outcome is very encouraging. Evidence in adults suggests that bleomycin is necessary for high cure rates in the majority of patients. In paediatrics, it appears unnecessary to use a weekly schedule of bleomycin, which is undoubtedly associated with a higher risk of lung toxicity. Moreover, the use of carboplatin may reduce the synergistic toxicity of cisplatin nephrotoxicity and bleomycin toxicity.

As discussed above, a relevant staging system is needed that would facilitate studies to determine which children are really low risk in whom bleomycin may be omitted and in whom carboplatin can be confidently used.

Box 17.1 Calculation of the correct dose for carboplatin

Dose (mg) = Desired AUC × [GFR + (20 × SA)]

or

Dose (mg) = Desired AUC × [GFR + (0.36 × weight)]

where GFR is the glomerular filtration rate (ml/min) and weight is body weight (kg).

Management of residual masses following chemotherapy

The management of residual masses following chemotherapy has received considered attention in adult practice, where even the presence of 'benign' teratoma following chemotherapy is associated with an increased risk of local recurrence. For this reason, where possible, surgery is recommended to remove any residual mass after chemotherapy. Examples of such residue are shown in Figures 17.5, 17.8 and 17.9. There is no indication for routine second-line chemotherapy simply because there is CT abnormality after six courses of primary chemotherapy. If a tumour is not resectable at this point then a biopsy is indicated to

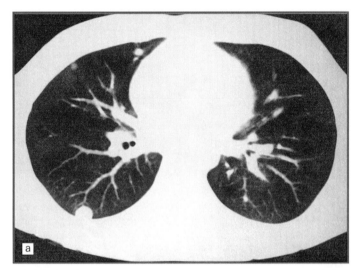

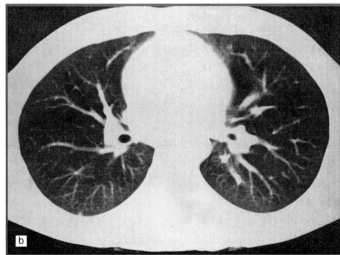

Figure 17.8 *Lung metastases at presentation (a) and at the end of six courses of PVB (b). A small subpleural lesion is evident at the end of treatment, which remained stable for 6 months and eventually disappeared with no further surgical or chemotherapy intervention.*

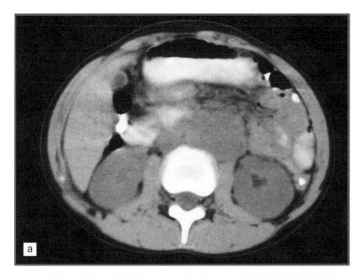

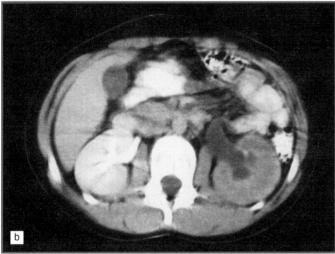

Figure 17.9 *Para-aortic nodal recurrence in a girl with ovarian GCT 6 months off treatment (a). There was an excellent response to second-line chemotherapy with IVAd (b) and she remains disease free.*

confirm whether viable undifferentiated tumour is present. If this is not the case, then a wait-and-watch policy with close monitoring of marker levels is appropriate. If there is evidence of residual undifferentiated tumour, then second-line chemotherapy is indicated (Fig. 17.9). At some sites in older children local radiotherapy may be more appropriate.

What second-line therapy should be used following relapse? Indications for second-line chemotherapy include:

- no decline in serum marker and an inoperable primary
- a clear increase in serum markers even if a partial response is seen at the primary site
- clinical relapse following cessation of chemotherapy.

Where the PVB, BEP or JEB regimen is used initially, second-line therapy should be with IVAd. There is ample evidence of activity for alkylating agents such as cyclophosphamide and ifosfamide and also doxorubicin. The standard IVAd with 9 g/m^2 ifosfamide is an active combination (Fig. 17.9). Alternatively, dose escalation with the Einhorn high-dose cisplatin/etoposide (200 mg/m^2 cisplatin) may be an effective strategy, although results with this have been somewhat disappointing.

Local radiotherapy is usually indicated only to consolidate second partial remission and depends upon the site of recurrent disease. For example, in a small infant with a recurrent sacrococcygeal tumour, intensified chemotherapy may be more appropriate than local radiotherapy.

What is the role of megatherapy? As in other highly chemosensitive tumours, dose escalation with agents known to be active in first-line treatment has been evaluated. Although there is little evidence in adults that dose escalation is effective as primary treatment in very high-risk patients, it may be an appropriate strategy where the likelihood of cure with second-line therapy is poor. Indications include:

- slow decline of markers with second-line chemotherapy
- to consolidate second complete remission where the primary tumour is unresectable and radiotherapy is to be avoided because of potential late sequelae
- incomplete first remission in patients with very bulky primary tumour where there has been slow marker decline or significant unresectable residual disease (Fig. 17.10).

The regimens used have generally been based on high-dose ifosfamide, carboplatin, etoposide and melphalan.

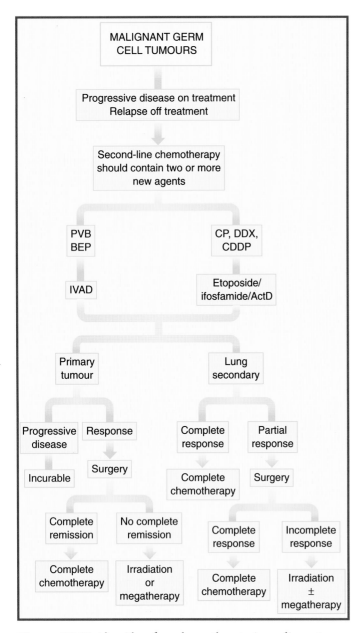

Figure 17.10 *Algorithm for salvage therapy in malignant germ cell tumours.*

Further reading

Hoffner, L., Deka, R., Chakravati, A. and Surti, U. (1994) Cytogenetics and origins of pediatric germ cell tumors. *Cancer Genetics and Cytogenetics* 74: 54–58.

Huddart, S.N., Mann, J.R., Gornall, P. *et al.* (1990) The UK Children's Cancer Study Group: testicular malignant germ cell tumours 1979–1988. *Journal of Pediatric Surgery* 25: 406–410.

Levi, J.A., Raghavan, D., Harvey, V. *et al.* (1993) The importance of bleomycin in combination chemotherapy for good-prognosis germ cell carcinoma. *Journal of Clinical Oncology* 11: 1300–1305.

Loehrer, P.J., Johnson, D., Elson, P. *et al.* (1995) Importance of bleomycin in favorable-prognosis disseminated germ cell tumors: an Eastern Cooperative Oncology Group trial. *Journal of Clinical Oncology* 13: 470–476.

Newell, D.R., Pearson, A.D.J., Balmanno, K. *et al.* (1993) Carboplatin pharmacokinetics in children: the development of a pediatric dosing formula. *Journal of Clinical Oncology* 11: 2314–2323.

Pinkerton, C.R., Pritchard, J. and Spitz, L. (1986) High complete response rate in children with advanced germ cell tumours using cisplatin-containing combination chemotherapy. *Journal of Clinical Oncology* 4: 194–199.

Pinkerton, C.R., Broadbent, V., Horwich, A. *et al.* (1990) JEB: a carboplatin based regimen for malignant germ cell tumours in children. *British Journal of Cancer* 62: 257–262.

Siegert, W., Beyer, J., Strohscheer, I. *et al.* (1994) High-dose treatment with carboplatin, etoposide and ifosfamide followed by autologous stem-cell transplantation in relapsed or refractory germ cell cancer: a phase I/II study. *Journal of Clinical Oncology* 12: 1223–1231.

Toner, G.C., Panicek, D.M., Heelan, R.T. *et al.* (1990) Adjunctive surgery after chemotherapy for nonseminomatous germ cell tumors: recommendations for patient selection. *Journal of Clinical Oncology* 8: 1683–1694.

Wheeler, B.M., Loehrer, P.J., Williams, S.D. *et al.* (1986) Ifosfamide in refractory male germ tumors. *Cancer* 4: 28–34.

Williams, S.D., Birch, R., Einhorn, L. *et al.* (1987) Treatment of disseminated germ cell tumors with cisplatin, bleomycin and either vinblastine or etoposide. *New England Journal of Medicine* 316: 1435–1440.

CHAPTER 18

Retinoblastoma

F. Doz and L. Desjardins

Introduction

Retinoblastoma is the most common ocular tumour in children, with an incidence of 1 in 15 000 to 20 000 births. Two-thirds of these tumours are unilateral and occur in children at a median age of 2 years at diagnosis. One-third of the tumours are hereditary and bilateral, with a median age of 1 year at diagnosis (Donaldson et al., 1997). This cancer, although curable for many years, still poses major problems in relation to several aspects:

- the prognosis related to the tumour itself: retinoblastoma is rarely a life-threatening disease in economically developed countries but remains a major concern in developing countries because of the frequency of metastatic and orbital extension
- the prognosis of patients suffering from hereditary forms of retinoblastoma who also have a genetic predisposition to other types of tumour: rarely, pinealoblastoma ('trilateral retinoblastoma') and, more frequently, secondary tumours, usually sarcomas
- visual prognosis: difficulties planning therapy that will allow eye preservation, and preservation of useful peripheral or central vision
- current limitations of genetic information given to the parents of affected children and to patients treated for retinoblastoma during childhood.

Some classical concepts concerning this disease have now become more complex. We will describe new

staging procedures, new therapeutic aspects, leading to revision of the indications for so-called 'reference' treatment, and some of the many genetic uncertainties, which often make counselling of affected families difficult or limited.

Staging procedure

The best staging procedure in intraocular disease is examination of the eye under general anaesthesia. This determines the size and location of the tumour(s), and the relationship between the tumour and the most important structures (fovea and the head of the optic nerve). The tumour should be clearly defined at diagnosis by drawings and clinical photographs. The Reese grouping is still useful but may be insufficient. It was designed to predict the chances of success of a conservative approach using external beam radiation therapy, but it does not take into account the difficulties of the treatment of posterior pole tumours when using new conservative techniques.

The examination under general anaesthesia must also be supplemented by an ultrasonographic examination of the eye, which is useful for measuring the size of the tumour(s) and evaluating further tumour response when a conservative treatment is indicated.

CT scan or MRI of the orbit and brain is mandatory for almost all patients but can be avoided in young children with small tumours that are not close to the optic disc. In these children, often diagnosed early because of a familial disease, the only staging procedure may be the examination of the eye and ultrasonography.

Other staging procedures have limited indications and are detailed in Figure 18.1 (Pratt *et al.*, 1989, 1990; Mohney and Robertson, 1994; Moscinski *et al.*, 1996; Karcioglu *et al.*, 1997).

Current therapeutic strategies

Adjuvant treatments after enucleation

The most common forms of retinoblastoma are unilateral. The diagnosis is usually established after tumour has spread, eliminating the possibility of conservative treatment (Fig. 18.2). The reference treatment in these unilateral forms is enucleation. Enucleation must be performed by a qualified surgeon following clear guidelines including:

* retaining sufficiently posterior section of the intraorbital optic nerve and preservation of all of the eye socket
* insertion of an implant that improves the quality of the subsequent prosthesis
* collection of tumour samples, in collaboration with the pathologist, for genetic studies.

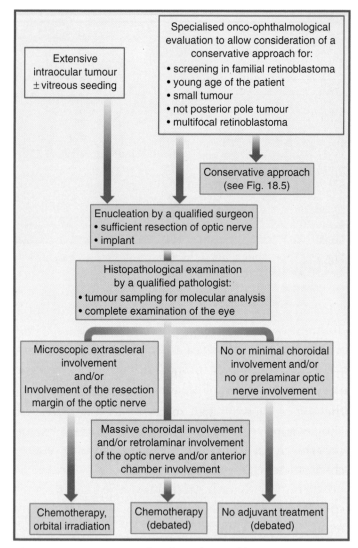

Figure 18.2 *Treatment of unilateral retinoblastoma.*

Histopathological examination must be performed by an experienced pathologist, examining the site of tumour spread in the retina, vitreous, choroid, sclera, optic nerve (by studying the relation with the cribriform plate and meninges) and the anterior chamber of the eye (Fig. 18.3). The degree of differentiation is also defined according to the abundance of 'rosette' cell groups, classically observed in neuro-ectodermal tumours. The histopathological study can define prognostic criteria indicating the need for adjuvant treatment after enucleation (Shields *et al.*, 1993, 1994; Khelfaoui *et al.*, 1996). Certain risk criteria have been clearly established: disruption of the sclera with microscopic invasion of the orbital soft tissues, invasion of the optic nerve resection margin. These forms require not only irradiation of the orbital cavity but also chemotherapy. The indications for adjuvant

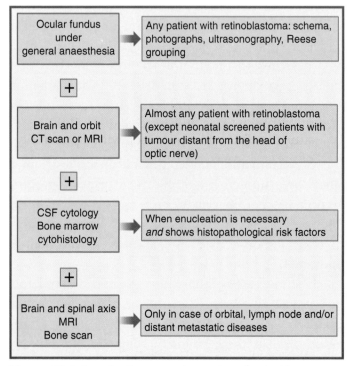

Figure 18.1 *Examinations to assist staging of retinoblastoma.*

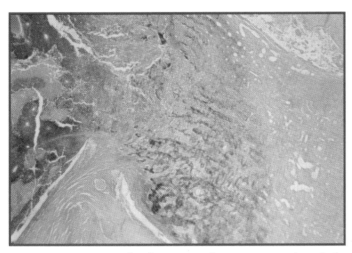

Figure 18.3 *Longitudinal section of an eye, enucleated for retinoblastoma. Retrolaminar involvement of retinoblastoma: group of basophil cells invade retina and vitreous (left), cross the cribriform plate (middle) and reach the retrolaminar part of the optic nerve (right).*

treatments for other forms of extraretinal invasion (isolated choroidal invasion, retrolaminar invasion of the optic nerve) are much more controversial (Kopelman *et al.*, 1987). These criteria, in our experience, still justify the use of postoperative chemotherapy (Khelfaoui *et al.*, 1996). A consensus has been reached that chemotherapy is necessary in the context of choroidal invasion associated with optic nerve invasion (Hungerford, 1993; Shields *et al.*, 1993). Ultimately, new laboratory prognostic criteria could prove useful for the future definition of adjuvant treatment indications (Doz *et al.*, 1996).

The drugs that are used in the adjuvant treatment of retinoblastoma are those which are active in other primitive neuro-ectodermal tumours: alkylating agents (cyclophosphamide), platinum compounds (carboplatin), vincristine, anthracyclines (adriamycin) and epipodophyllotoxins (etoposide) (White, 1991; Pratt *et al.*, 1994; Schwartzman *et al.*, 1996).

Treatment of orbital and metastatic forms

The objective of adjuvant treatment after enucleation is to prevent the development of orbital recurrence or metastases (metastases occur usually in bone, bone marrow and the CNS). The prognosis of these forms, considered until recently to be almost always fatal, has been improved by the use of new chemotherapy modalities and, maybe, high-dose chemotherapy with haematopoietic stem cell rescue (Doz and Pinkerton, 1994; Namouni *et al.*, 1997). Today, there is no standard treatment for extraocular retinoblastoma. The use of an intensive chemotherapy regimen may cure some patients with orbital disease (Doz *et al.*, 1994), lymph node metastases (Schwartzman *et al.*, 1996) and even distant metastatic disease (Namouni *et al.*, 1997). The prognosis of forms with CNS metastases, nevertheless, remains very poor. Embryonic tumours in the pineal gland (pinealoblastoma or 'trilateral retinoblastoma'), arising from optic vesicle cells (Kingston *et al.*, 1985; Blach *et al.*, 1994), can occur in the context of hereditary retinoblastomas and have a similar poor prognosis.

Conservative ocular treatments

Conservative treatments must be performed in specialised centres and are usually indicated in bilateral forms of retinoblastoma (Figs. 18.4 and 18.5). They can sometimes be indicated in unilateral form. Such situations include:

- diagnosis in the context of screening in patients with a family history of retinoblastoma: the tumour is often diagnosed at an early intraocular stage and, in this context, there is also a high risk of developing a metachronous lesion of the other eye
- young age at diagnosis: even in the absence of a family history, young age argues in favour of an hereditary form and, therefore, a risk of subsequent development of a tumour of the contralateral eye
- preservation of the functionally most important structures (macula, optic disc), with a possibility of preserving vision in affected eye.

The reference conservative treatment is external beam radiotherapy, which achieves tumour control in the great majority of patients (Donaldson *et al.*, 1997). However, increasingly frequently, its use should be limited in view of its late adverse effects such as:

- ophthalmological risks: the commonest risk is that of cataract, which can require subsequent surgical operations, as well as dry eye and photophobia, requiring tedious replacement

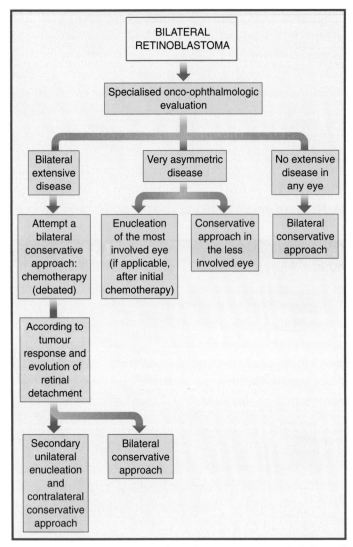

Figure 18.4 *Algorithm for the treatment of bilateral retinoblastoma.*

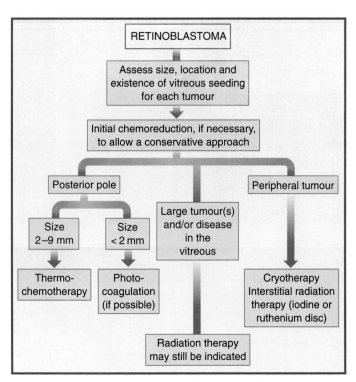

Figure 18.5 *Conservative approaches in retinoblastoma. At each step specialised onco-ophthalmological evaluation must occur.*

treatments. Other less common complications include keratitis, maculopathy, optic neuropathy, radiation retinopathy

- aesthetic effects: temporal bone undergrowth after use of a lateral beam is frequent, leading to facial asymmetry in the case of unilateral irradiation; use of an anterior beam for all or part of the irradiation carries a risk of palpebral retraction, loss of eyelashes and enophthalmos
- risk of pituitary irradiation (with, most importantly, subsequent growth hormone deficiency, possibly requiring replacement therapy) and, more rarely, depending on the technique used, a risk of brain irradiation and its long-term adverse effects

- major long-term risk in hereditary forms of retinoblastoma of predisposition to secondary sarcomas in the field of irradiation (Draper *et al.*, 1986). Irradiation actually potentiates the spontaneous predisposition associated with the constitutional anomaly of the RB1 gene.

Classical conservative ophthalmological treatments are highly effective but can generally only be used anterior to the equator of the eye. They consist of cryotherapy and radioactive iodine or ruthenium disc brachytherapy, avoiding any irradiation of the muscles and bones of the orbit. Photocoagulation can usually only be used in the posterior pole for tumours not exceeding 2 mm in diameter. In 1992, Murphree and co-workers described the use of thermochemotherapy for posterior pole tumours up to 9 mm in diameter (Murphree *et al.*, 1996). This treatment modality is based on the synergy between platinum-based chemotherapy, such as carboplatin, delivered by intravenous injection, and hyperthermia induced by a laser diode with a direct impact on the tumour (Fig. 18.6). This new technique has made posterior pole tumours even more often accessible to conservative treatments other than external beam radiotherapy (Murphree *et al.*, 1996; Levy *et al.*, 1998).

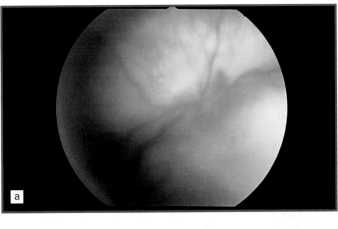

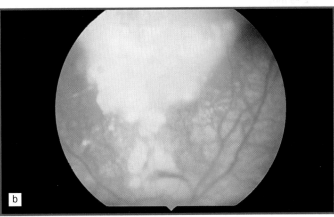

Figure 18.6 *Evolution towards cicatrisation of a posterior pole tumour treated with thermochemotherapy (systemic carboplatin chemotherapy followed by laser diode-induced tumoral hyperthermia). (a) Before treatment; (b) after treatment: tumour fragmentation and peripheral pigment.*

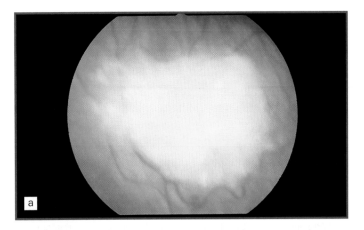

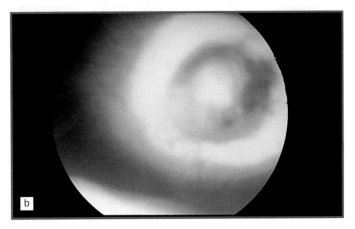

Figure 18.7 *Tumour response in a parapapillar tumour after two courses of chemotherapy with etoposide and carboplatin. (a) Before treatment; (b) after treatment: partial tumour fragmentation.*

Demonstration of the efficacy of chemotherapy in the rare forms of retinoblastoma with orbital involvement or metastases (Doz *et al.*, 1995) has also encouraged the use of 'neoadjuvant' chemotherapy for ocular tumours (Gallie *et al.*, 1996; Kingston *et al.*, 1996; Shields *et al.*, 1996; Levy *et al.*, 1998) with the following objectives:

- to make tumours accessible to conservative treatment in order to avoid enucleation
- to make tumours accessible to conservative treatment other than external beam radiotherapy
- to improve the visual prognosis of local conservative treatments by decreasing the territory of the retinal tumour and, sometimes, by decreasing macular and/or optic disc involvement.

The most frequently used drugs for neoadjuvant chemotherapy in the treatment of intraocular retinoblastoma are epipodophyllotoxins (etoposide more often than teniposide) associated with carboplatin (Fig. 18.7) and, for some authors, vincristine. The use of cyclosporin, combined with chemotherapy, has been described to improve tumour response and to increase the chance of success of a non-radiotherapeutic conservative treatment (Gallie *et al.*, 1996).

These new conservative treatment modalities must not mask two essential points:

- very extensive intraocular tumour does not appear to be accessible to conservative treatments other than external beam radiotherapy: all other conservative approaches are limited in terms of accessible tumour volume
- most anti-cancer drugs are potentially mutagenic and, in the context of hereditary retinoblastoma, the risk of an increased incidence of sarcoma by

the simple use of chemotherapy is not negligible (Jeha *et al.*, 1992; Winick *et al.*, 1993; Doz and Pinkerton, 1994).

Persistent genetic uncertainties

Retinoblastoma is a 'model' disease for the development of tumours caused by loss of an anti-oncogene. In the great majority of unilateral unifocal forms, the two anomalies of the RB1 gene are situated on retinal somatic cells. The other form (bilateral, unilateral multifocal) corresponds to a combination of a constitutional anomaly of the RB1 gene and a second event occurring on retinal somatic cells. The RB1 gene, situated at 13q1.4, has been cloned (Friend *et al.*, 1986) and analysis of its structure and expression in retinoblastoma has confirmed its anti-oncogene activity (Dunn *et al.*, 1989). Despite this detailed knowledge of the RB1 gene, genetic counselling of patients and their families remains difficult for a number of reasons:

- some unilateral unifocal forms are hereditary (Lohman *et al.*, 1997)
- even exhaustive analysis of the RB1 gene in clearly hereditary forms only reveals a causal constitutional anomaly of the RB1 gene in less than 30% of patients (Blanquet *et al.*, 1995; Lohman *et al.*, 1996)
- interpretation of anomalies detected on non-coding sequences of the RB1 gene still remains hazardous
- the RB1 gene mutation can occur at a late stage of embryogenesis, resulting in variable expression depending on the tissue. This mosaicism may prevent detection of the constitutional anomaly in blood lymphocytes
- penetrance is classically high, but rare spontaneously involuted forms ('retinomas') (Gallie *et al.*, 1982), or even skipped generations in hereditary forms, have been reported
- there is little established correlation between the type of genetic anomaly detected in the RB1 gene and the phenotypic course of the disease (Onadim *et al.*, 1992; Bremner *et al.*, 1997) and no established correlation with the development of second tumours

- exhaustive analyses of the RB1 gene are expensive and complex and, at the present time, cannot be performed routinely in all patients and their families.

Conclusions

Current therapeutic strategies of adjuvant chemotherapy after enucleation should be able to reduce the incidence of serious forms of retinoblastoma with orbital and metastatic involvement, which nevertheless remain frequent in developing countries. New therapeutic strategies of conservative treatment, avoiding external beam radiotherapy, tend to be more effective the smaller the intraocular tumour volume. It is, therefore, essential to promote retinoblastoma screening and early diagnosis by seriously considering symptoms reported by parents (leukocoria, strabismus), which are still all too frequently neglected.

Further reading

Blach, L.E., McCormick, B., Abramson, D.H. and Ellsworth, R.M. (1994) Trilateral retinoblastoma, incidence and outcome: a decade of experience. *International Journal of Radiation, Oncology, Biology and Physics* 29: 729–733.

Blanquet, V., Turleau, C., Gross-Morand, M.S. *et al.* (1995) Spectrum of germline mutations in the RB1 gene: a study of 232 patients with hereditary and non hereditary retinoblastoma. *Human Molecular Genetics* 4: 383–388.

Bremner, R., du Chan, D., Connoly-Wilson, M.J. *et al.* (1997) Deletion of RB exons 24 and 25 causes low-penetrance retinoblastoma. *American Journal of Human Genetics* 61: 556–570.

Donaldson, S., Egbert, P.R., Newsham, I. and Cavenee, W.K. (1997) Retinoblastoma. In *Principles and Practice of Pediatric Oncology*, 3rd edn. Pizzo P.A. and Poplack D.G., editors. Philadelphia, JB Lippincott, 1997: 699–716.

Doz, F. and Pinkerton, R. (1994) What is the place of carboplatin in paediatric oncology? *European Journal of Cancer* 30A: 194–201.

Doz, F., Khelfaoui, F., Mosseri, V. *et al.* (1994) The role of chemotherapy in orbital involvement of retinoblastoma: the experience of a single institution with 33 patients. *Cancer* 74: 722–732.

Doz, F., Neuenschwander, S., Plantaz, D. *et al.* (1995) Etoposide and carboplatin in extraocular retinoblastoma: a study by the Société Française d'Oncologie Pédiatrique. *Journal of Clinical Oncology* 13: 902–909.

Doz, F., Peter, M., Schleiermacher, G. *et al.* (1996) N-*myc* amplification, loss of heterozygosity on the short arm of chromosome 1 and DNA ploidy in retinoblastoma. *European Journal of Cancer* 32A: 645–649.

Draper, G.J., Sanders, B.M. and Kingston, J.E. (1986) Second primary neoplasms in patients with retinoblastoma. *British Journal of Cancer* 53: 661–671.

Dunn, J.M., Phillips, R.A., Becker, A.J. *et al.* (1989) Identification of germline and somatic mutations affecting the retinoblastoma gene. *Science* 241: 1797–1800.

Friend, S.H., Bernards, R., Rogelj, S. *et al.* (1986) A human DNA segment with properties of the gene that predisposes to retinoblastoma and osteosarcoma. *Nature* 323: 643–646.

Gallie, B.L., Ellsworth, L.M., Abramson, D.H. *et al.* (1982) Retinoma: spontaneous regression of retinoblastoma or benign manifestation of the mutation. *British Journal of Cancer* 45: 513–521.

Gallie, B., Budning, A., Deboer, G. *et al.* (1996) Chemotherapy with focal therapy can cure intraocular retinoblastoma without radiotherapy. *Archives in Ophthalmology* 114: 1321–1328.

Hungerford, J. (1993) Factors influencing metastasis in retinoblastoma. *British Journal of Ophthalmology* 77: 541.

Jeha, S., Jaffe, N. and Robertson, R. (1992) Secondary acute non-lymphoblastic leukemia in two children following treatment with a cis-diaminedichloroplatinum-II-based regimen for osteosarcoma. *Medical and Pediatric Oncology* 20: 71–74.

Karcioglu, Z.A., Al-Mesfer, S.A., Abboud, E. *et al.* (1997) Workup for metastatic retinoblastoma. A review of 261 patients. *Ophthalmology* 104: 307–312.

Khelfaoui, F., Validire, P., Auperin, A. *et al.* (1996) Histopathologic risk factors in retinoblastoma. A retrospective study of 172 patients treated in a single institution. *Cancer* 77: 1206–1213.

Kingston, J., Plowman, P. and Hungerford, J. (1985) Ectopic intracranial retinoblastoma in childhood. *British Journal of Ophthalmology* 69: 742–748.

Kingston, J.E., Hungerford, J.L. Madraperla, S.A. and Plowman, P.N. (1996) Results of combined chemotherapy and radiotherapy for advanced intraocular retinoblastoma. *Archives in Ophthalmology* 114: 1339–1343.

Kopelman, J.E., McClean, I.W. and Rosenberg, S.H. (1987) Multivariate analysis of risk factors for metastasis in retinoblastoma treated by enucleation. *Ophthalmology* 94: 371–377.

Levy, C., Doz, F., Quintana, E. *et al.* (1998) The role of chemotherapy alone or in combination with hyperthermia in the primary treatment of intraocular retinoblastoma: preliminary results in 30 patients treated at Institut Curie. *British Journal of Ophthalmology*, in press.

Lohman, D.R., Brandt, B., Hopping, W. *et al.* (1996) The spectrum of RB1 germline mutations in hereditary retinoblastoma. *American Journal of Human Genetics* 58: 940–949.

Lohman, D., Gerick, M., Brandt, B. *et al.* (1997) Constitutional RB1-gene mutations in patients with isolated unilateral retinoblastoma. *American Journal of Human Genetics* 61: 282–294.

Mohney, B.G. and Robertson, D.M. (1994) Ancillary testing for metastasis in patients with newly diagnosed retinoblastoma. *American Journal of Ophthalmology* 118: 707–711.

Moscinski, L.C., Pendergrass, T.W., Weiss, A. *et al.* (1996) Recommendations for the use of routine bone marrow aspiration and lumbar punctures in the follow-up of patients with retinoblastoma. *Journal of Pediatric Hematology and Oncology* 18: 130–134.

Murphree, A.L., Villablanca, J.G., Deegan, W.F. *et al.* (1996) Chemotherapy plus local treatment in the management of intraocular retinoblastoma. *Archives of Ophthalmology* 114: 1348–1356.

Namouni, F., Doz, F., Tanguy, M.L. *et al.* (1997) High dose chemotherapy with carboplatin, etoposide and cyclophosphamide followed by hematopoietic stem cell rescue in patients with high risk retinoblastoma: a SFOP and SFGM study. *European Journal of Cancer* 33: 2368–2375.

Onadim, Z., Hogg, A., Baird, P.N. and Cowell, J.K. (1992) Oncogenic point mutations in exon 20 of the RB1 gene in families showing incomplete penetrance and mild expression of the retinoblastome phenotype. *Proceedings of the National Academy of Sciences of the USA* 89: 6177–6181.

Pratt, C.B., Meyer, D., Chenaille, P. and Crom D.B. (1997) The use of bone marrow aspirations and lumbar punctures at the time of diagnosis of retinoblastoma. *Journal of Clinical Oncology* 7: 140–143.

Pratt, C.B., Crom, D.B., Magill, L. *et al.* (1990) Skeletal scintigraphy in patients with bilateral retinoblastoma. *Cancer* 65: 26–28.

Pratt, C.B., Fontanesi, J., Chenaille, P. *et al.* (1994) Chemotherapy for extraocular retinoblastoma. *Pediatric Hematology and Oncology* 11: 301–309.

Schwartzman, E., Chantada, G., Fandino, A. *et al.* (1996) Results of a stage-based protocol for the treatment of retinoblastoma. *Journal of Clinical Oncology* 14: 1532–1536.

Shields, C.L., Shields, J.A., Baez, K. *et al.* (1993) Choroidal invasion of retinoblastoma: metastatic potential and clinical risk factor. *British Journal of Ophthalmology* 77: 544–548.

Shields, C.L., Shields, J.A., Baez, K. *et al.* (1994) Optic nerve invasion of retinoblastoma. Metastatic potential and clinical risk factors. *Cancer* 73: 692–698.

Shields, C., de Potter, P., Himelstein, B. *et al.* (1996) Chemoreduction in the initial management of intraocular retinoblastoma. *Archives in Ophthalmology* 114: 1330–1338.

White, L. (1991) Chemotherapy in retinoblastoma: current status and future directions. *American Journal of Pediatric Hematology and Oncology* 13: 189–201.

Winick, N.J., McKenna, R.W., Shuster, J.J. *et al.* (1993) Secondary acute myeloid leukemia in children with acute lymphoblastic leukemia treated with etoposide. *Journal of Clinical Oncology* 11: 209–217.

Index